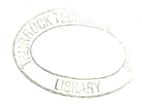

A HANDBOOK FOR
ASTHMA SELF-MANAGEMENT:
A LEADER'S GUIDE TO
LIVING WITH ASTHMA

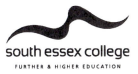

south essex college

FURTHER & HIGHER EDUCATION

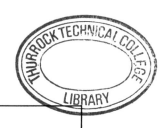

A HANDBOOK FOR ASTHMA SELF-MANAGEMENT: A LEADER'S GUIDE TO LIVING WITH ASTHMA

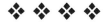

Thomas L. Creer

Harry Kotses

Russ V. Reynolds

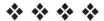

Ohio University Press
Athens

Ohio University Press books are printed on acid-free paper ∞

LIBRARY OF CONGRESS CATALOGING-IN-PUBLICATION DATA
Creer, Thomas L.
         A handbook for asthma self-management : a leader's guide to living
with asthma / Thomas L. Creer, Harry Kotses, Russ V. Reynolds.
      p.   cm.
      Includes bibliographical references (p.)
      ISBN 0-8214-0990-5 (pbk.)   ~ 616.238
      1. Asthma–Patients –Rehabilitation. 2. Self-help groups.
I. Kotses, Harry. II. Reynolds, Russ V. III. Title.
RC591.C74 1991b   90-21146
616.2'3803–dc20   CIP

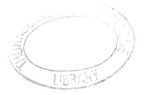

TABLE OF CONTENTS

INTRODUCTION TO A LEADER'S GUIDE FOR
A HANDBOOK FOR ASTHMA SELF-MANAGEMENT

PHILOSOPHY OF THE ASTHMA SELF-MANAGEMENT PROGRAM

Asthma Self-Management is based upon the following premises:

1. Patients can play a significant role in the management of their asthma.

2. Being knowledgeable about asthma is a prerequisite for self-management.

3. Self-management skills performed by patients are an integral part of asthma management.

4. Self-management skills can be taught to patients with asthma.

5. Patients benefit from contact with other asthmatic patients. They share experiences and common concerns, and teach each other effective methods for managing asthma and the consequences of the disorder.

6. Patients can become allies with their physicians and other health care personnel in the management of asthma.

PHILOSOPHY OF SELF-MANAGEMENT

Kanfer (1980) described 12 features that are incorporated into most effective self-management programs (Table I:1). Where possible, these were integrated into Asthma Self-Management. Since each group of patients will differ from one another, it is imperative that leaders be aware of the 12 features and introduce them where and when it is appropriate to do so. The 12 features require that you:

1. Continually attend to the concerns of patients. While most topics will be covered through the format provided by Asthma Self-Management, any given group of patients is apt to raise questions that have not been asked before. By carefully listening to participants, the group leader can detect and address these questions. Also, by asking patients how they solve specific asthma-related problems, the leader can learn about approaches he or she may wish to incorporate into later sessions with other participants.

2. Be certain that the patients are observing and monitoring the key target behaviors required to successfully manage their asthma. No matter how long patients are involved with a program, it is essential that these checks be made.

3. Develop a plan for changing the patients' behavior. The acquisition and performance of the self-management skills taught in Asthma Self-Management usually encompass all areas of relevant behavior change necessary to successfully manage asthma. However, by attending to the comments of individual patients, you can target other problem behaviors that require individual attention.

TABLE I:1. TWELVE FEATURES OF
EFFECTIVE SELF-MANAGEMENT PROGRAMS
(Kanfer, 1980)

Attend to concerns of patients

Be certain patients attend to target behavior

Develop plan to change patients' behaviors

Describe assumptions and rationales underlying
 self-management skills

Model and role play desired behaviors

Verify patients' progress and provide feedback to them

Record and inspect quantitative and qualitative data
 obtained from patients

Employ reinforcement

Assess patients' performance of self-management
 behaviors in natural environment

Describe self-management skills, when and how they
 should be applied, and the type of data to be collected

Provide strong support

Constantly summarize and reiterate key concepts

4. Describe to patients the assumptions and rationale underlying each self-management skill. Many of these skills will be easily recognizable to most patients; however, there are other skills, such as proper use of a peak flow meter, that may require an explanation.

5. Model and role play desired behaviors for patients. For example, you might model the proper use of the peak flow meter to ensure patients correctly use the instrument.

6. Verify patients' progress and provide feedback to patients about their performance. This process must become an integral part of all patient contacts; the feedback not only can correct any problems, but it also provides reinforcement to patients.

7.   Record and inspect quantitative and qualitative data obtained from patients that document any behavioral changes or the performance of self-management skills. This must also be a function that you regularly perform in contacts with patients.

8.   Employ a reinforcement system that gradually shifts from the reinforcement provided by you and others to self-reinforcement provided by the patients for their successful self-management of their asthma. The latter process requires that they use appropriate standards for self-evaluation of performance and self-management outcomes.

9.   Assess whether patients execute any newly-acquired behaviors in the natural environment. If required, you may need to discuss and make additional suggestions to patients to insure that behavior change generalizes from thought to action and from the clinic to day-to-day living.

10. Frequently describe self-management skills, when and how they should be applied, and the type of data you wish collected by the patients. Reiteration of key skills is useful to patients.

11. Provide strong support to patients for their accepting increased responsibility for the care and management of their asthma. In addition, provide support for their continuing to perform self-management skills over the duration of the program.

12. Constantly summarize and reiterate key concepts involved in the self-management of asthma. This entails the summarization of self-management skills, as well as the application of these skills to new asthma-related problems and situations.

MOTIVATIONAL APPROACHES TO TAKE IN TEACHING SELF-MANAGEMENT SKILLS TO PARTICIPANTS

Kanfer & Schefft (1988) have suggested 20 motivational approaches that can be used in teaching self-management skills (Table I-2). The relevance of each step in teaching self-management skills to asthmatic adults is as follows:

1.   **Disrupting automatic responses.** Asthmatic patients often have approaches to treating their asthma, such as waiting for the attack to intensify enough so that it requires treatment at a hospital emergency room. These represent automatic responses on the part of the patients. Your task is to teach self-management skills to permit participants to develop a new perspective on the treatment of asthma. This may take the form of their "reframing" the way they consider attacks in order to treat them in a more effective and economical manner.

2.   **Encouraging use of self-regulation skills.** These skills form the backbone of the self-management of asthma.

3.   **Making small demands.** At first, participants may feel overwhelmed in learning the role self-management can play in the future control of their asthma. For this reason, Asthma Self-Management has been prepared to teach participants to accept and achieve limited objectives within a reasonable period of time. These are scaled down further by the pattern of review and repetition of key concepts throughout the program.

TABLE I:2. MOTIVATIONAL APPROACHES FOR TEACHING SELF-MANAGEMENT SKILLS
(Kanfer & Shefft, 1988)

Disrupting automatic responses

Encouraging use of self-regulation skills

Making small demands

Doing something associated with a task

Doing a task without fear of failure

Associating outcomes with previous reinforcers

Re-attributing causes

Using role play

Working towards self-generated goals

Using "provocative strategies"

Encouraging positive self-reinforcement

Recording progress

Using environmental cues

Requiring a prior commitment

Making contracts

Promoting a facilitative program

Using the therapeutic alliance

Using seeding

Encouraging patients to dream new dreams

Being enthusiastic and supportive

4. **Doing something associated with a task.** The use of homework assignments, such as those presented in the patient's guide, permits participants to learn self-management skills. By doing so, participants can learn weekly tasks which facilitate changing their manner of managing their asthma.

5. **Doing a task without fear of failure.** Asthma Self-Management has been designed to attain patient success in the management of the disorder. There may be limits to self-management in controlling all attacks, but participants must never fear that their actions will lead to failure. It is the omission of the performance of self-management skills that produces failure.

6. **Associating outcomes with previous reinforcers.** A component of Asthma Self-Management is to review weekly how participants applied their self-management skills to control attacks. This performance, when successful, is reinforcing to participants. In addition, reinforcement by group leaders and other members of the group strengthens participants' performance.

7. **Re-attributing causes.** Re-attributing the causes of problems from the patient's inability to his or her insufficient effort or to factors not under their control can increase the participant's persistence and effort in performing self-management skills. Re-attribution can also reduce a patient's fear of engaging in a change program.

8. **Using role play.** A number of problems are presented to participants to solve. Patients may wish to use role playing in arriving at potential solutions to these problems.

9. **Working toward self-generated goals.** Asthma Self-Management is designed to teach patients to set goals for themselves in the management of their asthma. In conjunction with their physicians, it is hoped that participants can generate more and more realistic goals as they progress through the program.

10. **Using "provocative strategies."** These strategies are not built into Asthma Self-Management. However, many patients have experienced problems in the management of their asthma, which have led them to seek to establish self-control over their disorder. These experiences will be shared in all groups who participate in Asthma Self-Management; it is up to the group leader to apply these strategies to motivate all participants.

11. **Encouraging positive self-reinforcement.** Participants must be taught to use self-reinforcement skills when they successfully apply self-management skills to help manage their asthma. This approach is highlighted throughout Asthma Self-Management.

12. **Recording progress.** The use of asthma diaries and report-of-attack forms presented in the patient's guide, permits patients to chart their progress; such information is not only of use to you, but it provides positive feedback to the participants.

13. **Using environmental cues.** Environmental cues, such as a pill container that signals when medications are to be taken, can assist patients to better control their asthma. Other environmental cues, such as stimuli that can trigger attacks, become part of the perceptions and subsequent action taken by patients involved with Asthma Self-Management. Environmental stimuli that trigger attacks are listed in the patient's guide.

14. **Requiring a prior commitment.** It is important that when the program is explained to them, participants make the commitment to enter into the Asthma Self-Management Program. Without such a commitment, they are unlikely either to complete the program or to perform the skills taught in Asthma Self-Management.

15. **Making contracts.** When patients decide to enroll in Asthma Self-Management, there is an implied contract that they will make every effort to attend all sessions, complete assigned homework, and practice self-management skills. Without this implied contract, there remains a question about a participant's commitment to the program.

16. **Promoting a facilitative program.** As noted throughout this manual, a role of the leader is to promote a program that is facilitative to the acquisition of self-management skills. Such an environment also permits patients to share their experiences, as well as to make suggestions that all can use in managing future attacks.

17. **Using the therapeutic alliance.** The relationship that is formed by participants, both with the group leader and with other members of the group, can promote and maintain change.

18. **Using seeding.** "Seeding" is a term used to describe the preparation of patients for the future discussion of other topics in the self-management of asthma. This approach is taken at the end of each session in Asthma Self-Management both in assigning homework and in briefly describing what will occur during the next session.

19. **Encouraging patients to dream new dreams.** This entails teaching participants to imagine new ways they can apply the self-management skills they have been taught. Whereas patients may only perform some skills in specific situations, the range of settings will expand so that, over the course of their participation, they begin to develop ways to use their skills across a wide array of contexts.

20. **Be enthusiastic and supportive.** A major ingredient for the success of Living With Asthma for Children and Parents was the enthusiasm and support both of the group leaders and of participants. This made a significant difference in motivating participants to learn and perform the self-management skills they were taught in the program; the same component is essential for Asthma Self-Management.

ORGANIZATION OF GROUP LEADER'S GUIDE

The group leader materials for each session include a session overview, activity outline, teaching notes, background reading, references, and visuals.

1. SESSION OVERVIEW: This includes a list of session goals, as well as the equipment or supplies required for the session.

2. ACTIVITY OUTLINE: The major teaching/learning events are listed, with notes about the materials required for each topic, as well as the suggested time allotted for each section.

3. **TEACHING NOTES:** These provide detailed instructions for conducting the sessions. The notes serve two important purposes: (a) They summarize the content of the material to be covered; and (b) provide stylistic suggestions about methods of presentation.

4. **BACKGROUND READING:** Recent research findings and background material have been summarized so group leaders can begin to develop a knowledge base about the behavioral and medical management of asthma.

5. **REFERENCES:** This enumerates the references to materials summarized in the background readings.

6. **VISUALS:** A series of visual materials, designed for use with an overhead projector, have been prepared for each session. These describe key concepts of the program and help organize the group leader's presentation.

TEACHING THE SESSIONS

The optimal number of group participants is 6 to 12 adult patients. It is difficult to permit free and open discussion by all participants in groups larger than twelve. Fewer than six participants can limit the opportunity for discussion and feedback.

The atmosphere of the sessions must be informal. All participants should be encouraged to become actively involved. They must feel free to ask questions, express their feelings, share experiences, make comments, and develop solutions to problems. From the outset, emphasize that there is no such thing as a dumb question; participants should feel free to make any comments that they wish to make. As underscored throughout the program, a goal of the Asthma Self-Management program is to help participants integrate self-management skills into their daily lives.

While free expression is encouraged, it is important to prevent two unwanted situations . First, no single individual should dominate the conversation throughout the program. During the initial sessions of the program, one person can make a contribution by speaking more than others. Later, however, such conversation may lead others not to speak up. It is the task of the moderator to reduce the input from one individual by having others share their experiences and concerns. Sometimes direct feedback to the dominating participant, outside of the group sessions, is necessary. Second, all participants should, by the end of the program, be contributing to the program. It is often the person who speaks very little at the outset who later has the most profound insights into asthma and its management. Encourage everyone to share their unique perspectives and experiences.

A variety of teaching methods are used in Asthma Self-Management. They include:

1. Lectures, handouts (contained in the client manual), and question-and-answer sessions;

2. Readings, explanations, problem-solving techniques, audiotapes, and guided participation
in learning how to relax; and,

3. Discussion, idea sharing, and, from the very first session, practice in making decisions to solve problems typically faced by patients with asthma.

At the beginning of the program, the leader assumes the role of a lecturer. Most of the didactic material is presented in the initial two sessions. With the passage of sessions, however, the leader becomes a facilitator of group discussion. This occurs because all participants will wish to contribute to the discussion; the role of the leader thus becomes one of directing the session so that everyone has the opportunity to express their ideas and experiences. It is common for the leader to learn as much from the participants as they do from the leader.

When participants arrive for a weekly meeting, it is an ideal time to review any of their data for which you have questions. If data is missing on the asthma diary, for example, it is easy for you to ask a participant to provide you with any missing information before the start of the session. Be certain to greet each participant by name and, if time permits, to answer any lingering questions that may have arisen during an earlier session or to ask them about anything that may have occurred with their asthma in the preceding week. To answer patient questions may require that you contact someone other than a member of your project staff. This is not difficult, but it may require that you visit a medical library or contact an expert, such as an allergist or chest physician.

Provide refreshments and snacks throughout each meeting. If the group wishes, take a 5- or 10-minute midsession break to permit participants to obtain a refreshment, go to the restroom, etc. This time can also permit you to converse with a co-leader with respect to the direction you wish to go during the remainder of the time. Usually, however, adults are not especially interested in formal breaks. They generally obtain whatever refreshment they wish during or after the session. Plan on remaining 15 minutes or more after a session because participants often remain to discuss various topics.

Refer to the client manual when discussing homework assignments. Between session homework includes readings in the client manual and various worksheets contained in the appendix of the client manual.

FOSTERING POSITIVE GROUP DYNAMICS

GROUP LEADER SKILLS

Many of the principles and procedures outlined in *Living With Asthma for Children and Parents*, (Creer, Backial, Ullman & Leung, 1986) have been synthesized into Asthma Self-Management. Both programs are likely to be effective if group leaders adhere to the following guidelines:

1. Actively listen to all participants;

2. Maintain eye contact with participants when they are talking to either the leader or to another member of the group;

3. Thoroughly review the necessary background material for each session;

4. Seek clarification when needed and admit to a lack of knowledge when appropriate (the treatment of asthma is truly an interdisciplinary effort and group leaders are not expected to be experts in all areas);

6. Actively seek involvement of all participants in the discussion; however, the leader cannot force anyone to participate; and,

7. Know when to exercise restraint and allow the group to come to its own realizations and understanding.

Other facets of group leader behavior can enhance group development. Personal characteristics of warmth, empathy, and genuineness help set the tone for the entire program. This promotes communication among members of the group. Second, the leader can appropriately share personal experiences to illustrate what is taught to participants. The more conversant the leader is with both factual information and anecdotes about asthma, the more likely he or she will relate to each participant. Third, the leader must foster simultaneous loose-tight properties in the meetings. Although open discussion is encouraged, the leader must also be certain that key concepts of any given session are covered. There are specific asthma knowledge and self-management skills to be taught to participants in each session. It is tempting to drift and discuss topics of interest to the group, such as medication side-effects or the characteristics of individual physicians. Attend to and avoid these sirens of distraction; they can defeat the purpose of any particular session. Finally, the leader must perceive the group as an entity to itself and proceed with the interest of the group in mind. For example, forfeit discussing a favorite topic or subject if it is not relevant to the group at hand.

Usually by the second or third session of Asthma Self-Management, group cohesion has begun to occur. The group leader will know this has happened when group members become supportive and understanding of their fellow participants, and when they open up and talk comfortably. They begin to feel that they can laugh at themselves, and they recognize their own shortcomings and need for improvement. The guidelines offered in this discussion will help establish strong group rapport.

To foster group rapport, a number of suggestions are offered (Table I:3):

1. Point out the commonality of the participants' experiences; this will help build cohesiveness among group members. As they realize that they share common experiences, several types of comments can help to foster links among group members:

    a. Who else has experienced similar reactions or feelings?

    b. What has been your experience with the problem?

    c. Have any of the other participants observed such experiences?

    d. How has anyone else dealt with a similar situation?

2. Remind the group that they already have learned much about asthma management through their everyday experience. Their efforts in the program will be to refine and add to what they have learned.

3. Encourage participants to trust their own experiences. Do not hesitate to share your experiences with asthma or to describe stories and solutions offered by members of other asthma self-management groups you have taught. Group leader self-disclosure is appropriate if it is relevant to the group or material being covered; beware of sharing experiences that are not directly related to the group. The group is usually more willing to open up if you do so first. Less personal disclosure may be needed once the group members openly share among themselves. At this time, the leader can rely on the group for generating personal experiences. Encourage participants to help each other as well.

TABLE I:3. TIPS FOR FOSTERING GROUP RAPPORT

Emphasize commonality of the patients' experiences

Emphasize previous acquisition of knowledge of
  asthma management

Encourage patients to trust their own experiences

Trust the group

Establish and maintain the idea that it is the patients' group

Use positive social reinforcement

Greet each participant by name before and during
  each session

---

4. Trust the group. Allow them to choose the direction of discussion as long as it remains within the range set by the topic. Remember the loose-tight qualities of the session that you wish to attain. You may need to redirect the group if they are floundering, but do not force them to move in any particular direction. You may need to redefine the nature and purpose of the group if some participants dominate to the detriment of other members. Direct feedback outside of the group session may be helpful.

5. Establish and maintain the idea that it is the participants' group. In order for them to have a positive experience, it is vital that they feel they can learn from each other. At the beginning, one or two members of the group may talk more than others; there will be several, in fact, who may say little, if anything, during the first or second session. As the sessions progress, be certain that one or two members do not dominate the discussion, but that everyone contributes. This state is usually not difficult to achieve; there are no patients with asthma who are neutral about the disorder.

6. Use positive social reinforcement. Reinforce participants for coming on time, for asking questions, for following up on issues with their physicians, for trying new ideas, and for attempting to work out problems.

7. As participants assemble at the start of each session, try to greet each person who comes in. This helps participants feel welcome and accepted. Try to talk to each person, but do not engage in lengthy conversations with any one at the exclusion of others. Later in the program, other group members will begin to greet their fellow participants and ask them about their week. Congratulate the group when you see that the group has started to discuss and solve many asthma-related problems.

OTHER CONSIDERATIONS IN CONDUCTING ASTHMA SELF-MANAGEMENT

1. Continually stress the goals of the program.

2. Reinforce participants when they report they are performing self-management skills.

3. Reinforce, by describing what occurred to the entire group, when a participant handles a particularly difficult problem in an appropriate manner.

4. Stress that being a good health-care consumer is integral to good self-management.

5. Be knowledgeable about the topics to be discussed in each session. Not only read the materials that are presented in the leader's guide, but also the client materials on each topic. You may also wish to do additional readings on any of the material covered; the background readings in the group guide often are followed by a reference list of relevant sources.

6. Whenever participants ask specific questions about their asthma and its treatment, ask them to review these questions with their physicians. Check at the next meeting that the participants have followed through on this action.

LEADING QUESTIONS AND RESPONSES

The following questions and comments have been helpful in guiding and prompting group discussion. The leading phrases can be integrated into any of the sessions; responses to the questions can be helpful in maintaining a positive tone in the discussions.

GROUP LEADER QUESTIONS

How would you handle that problem?

Do any of you have any questions or comments?

Has anyone here experienced a similar problem? If you did, how did you handle it?

Have any of you heard of similar problems and how were they handled?

Does it all sound familiar?

Is anyone surprised by that?

Are there any skills you've learned thus far which you think would be helpful in managing the problem?

Do you believe you could handle a similar problem?

GROUP LEADER ANSWERS

"I think I see what you are saying."--This is a useful way of acknowledging someone's statement without agreeing or disagreeing with it.

"That's a good point."--This reinforces the person for making the statement. Use oral rewards liberally throughout all sessions. Other encouraging gestures, such as a nod, are also effective in reinforcing statements made by members of the group.

"Let me see if I've got this straight."--With this statement, you may wish to essentially repeat what the person has said to you. This clarifies the comment for you and other members of the group. The practice is particularly useful when the patient has made a good point and you think it bears repeating so that all group members understand what was said.

"Let me summarize for the group what you have said."--This provides you the opportunity to summarize several comments by a participant in a manner that makes the issue clear to other members of the group.

"I'm not certain that I understand what you are saying."--Don't be afraid to ask a participant to clarify his or her statement; this not only improves communication, but permits the entire group to share in what is said.

"That's a good point. Let me see if I can put it within the framework of what we have been learning in this class."--Never miss the opportunity to place remarks by participants, when they are appropriate, within the context of the Asthma Self-Management program. This is an excellent way to reinforce participants.

"That's an excellent question, but I don't think I can answer it completely. Give me a week to obtain the answer for you."--When you don't have an answer, respond honestly. It is important to follow through with your promise of an answer during the next session as the participant's trust in you may depend upon it.

IMPLEMENTING ASTHMA SELF-MANAGEMENT

THE SETTING

The requirements for conducting a program are simple: a meeting room with a large table and enough chairs for everyone to sit comfortably; a place to display visuals; and a place for refreshments. Such rooms are commonly found in hospitals, clinics, schools, or churches. It does not matter where the sessions are conducted as long as informal interaction can occur among participants and between participants and staff. Two of the sessions, in which relaxation exercises are introduced, require that reclining chairs or bedrolls (for the floor) be available.

SPONSORING ORGANIZATIONS

Any number of organizations may sponsor an Asthma Self-Management program. Hospitals, community health centers, local chapters of the American Lung Association, health maintenance organizations, group practices, schools, and state or local health departments are likely sponsors. Local medical societies, employee medical programs, or health insurers may also wish to sponsor programs.

WHO CAN TEACH THE SESSIONS?

Thus far, those involved in teaching Asthma Self-Management include psychologists, nurses, health care specialists, health educators, and physicians. However, the program has been designed to be taught by others, including those who have previously participated in the program, respiratory therapists, school nurses, school health educators, physicians' assistants, nurse practitioners, or other health personnel.

We have previously described what is necessary to successfully teach Asthma Self-Management. These include: (a) a thorough knowledge of asthma and self-management principles; (b) a sensitivity to the problems of patients with asthma; (c) characteristics of warmth, empathy, and genuineness; and (d) an ability to lead and facilitate group discussion (Table I:4). Prior experience with small group process is helpful. However, a potential leader can learn these skills by participating in the program and reading books about group dynamics and discussion facilitation methods. Many health care practitioners are well-versed in conducting such groups; thus, they should feel confident in applying what is taught in the two manuals that comprise Asthma Self-Management.

TABLE I:4. SKILLS REQUIRED FOR TEACHING ASTHMA SELF-MANAGEMENT TO ADULTS

Thorough knowledge of asthma and self-management techniques

Sensitivity to problems of asthmatic patients

Characteristics of warmth, empathy, and genuineness

Ability to lead and facilitate group discussion

RECRUITMENT OF PARTICIPANTS

A number of techniques have been used to recruit participants for Asthma Self-Management for adults. These include:

1. **Personal letters to physicians**. Personal letters to physicians that explain the program can be a helpful first step in enrolling participants in Asthma Self-Management. However, the number of referrals is likely to be low unless these letters are followed up by a personal contact with the physician.

2. **Talks before local medical groups and societies**. It is important to explain to physicians that self-management programs are not a threat to their practice, but that they offer a way to augment sound medical treatment. Through the application of self-management skills, patients do become allies with their physicians. Although there may be little immediate response at such meetings, they are useful in recruiting participants if followed by one-on-one contacts with medical personnel.

3. **Visits with the staff at local health maintenance organizations (HMOs).** The responses of personnel at HMOs are variable. There are many who view the programs as useful in reducing costs. These staff generally will refer patients to programs such as Asthma Self-Management. There are personnel at other HMOs,

however, who, for various reasons, are not enthusiastic about such programs. The best sources of referrals are from physicians who voluntarily participate in HMOs or other physician-controlled health maintenance plans. These physicians realize that both they and their patients can benefit if their patients develop self-management skills. The physicians are aware that patients can manage many problems for which they formerly contacted their physicians; by doing so, the physicians can focus on difficult cases that require more of their attention. Patients, on the other hand, become partners with their physician in the management of their disorder. Thus, effective asthma management is beneficial to both physicians and their patients.

4. **Visits with the staff at community health care centers and hospitals.** The staff at these facilities are usually enthusiastic about having their patients participate in Asthma Self-Management. Since most health care systems are stretched thin by high patient volume and limited budgets, having patients shoulder more responsibility for their health care is received with open arms. Most such centers make every effort to help enroll patients into the program. However, the patients show varying degrees of motivation about their involvement in such programs. A few are enthusiastic: They realize their participation offers an opportunity for them to take greater control over their health. Other participants, however, are less motivated: They will visit a nearby health center during times of crisis, but tend to miss appointments and are noncompliant when asthma-free. It requires considerable time and tolerance to recruit and maintain the involvement of these patients.

5. **Community announcements.** Public service announcements on radio and television can help recruit participants for Asthma Self-Management. Newspaper articles or advertisements describing the program are also effective in the recruitment of participants. Many who respond to such announcements follow through and become involved in Asthma Self-Management. Public service announcements often reach patients who would otherwise not have heard of the program.

   There are two major problems that can occur with public service announcements. First, people will respond who do not have asthma or, second, who want financial remuneration for participating in the program. For this reason, careful screening must occur to eliminate those who do not have asthma or who have other motives for wishing to participate. You should insist that potential participants have their own physicians so that a partnership between patients and their physicians can be fostered through participation in Asthma Self-Management.

   Community announcements should contain a specific description of Asthma Self-Management. A sample news fact sheet is presented at the end of the introduction. Use this as a guideline in preparing materials to be sent to newspapers or radio and television stations. There are usually designated persons at newspaper or radio and television stations, be it a lifestyle, health, or local news editors, who can assist you with information about the necessary lead time and preparation of any public service.

6. **Descriptive flyers.** The purpose of these flyers is twofold. First, they describe the basics of the program to potential participants. Second, the flyers save time and effort on the part of physicians and other health care personnel who wish to publicize the program. Copies of these flyers can be left in the waiting rooms of clinics and hospitals. In addition, they can be placed on the bulletin boards of churches, businesses, and

community centers. We have found it especially useful to keep a stack of the flyers in the emergency rooms of hospitals. By doing so, asthmatic patients and their families can read the flyer when they are most apt to seek participation in the program.

ADDITIONAL STEPS IN SETTING UP THE ASTHMA SELF-MANAGEMENT PROGRAM

After an agency or group has agreed to sponsor Asthma Self-Management and the process of recruiting participants has begun, several other steps remain:

1. **Designate a contact person for the group.** Usually, the leader of the group is the contact person. However, it may be that a staff member of the sponsoring agency can assume this role. The name of this person and his or her telephone number should be listed on the flyer. This way, the prospective participant knows who to call for information regarding Asthma Self-Management.

2. **Secure a meeting room for all of the sessions.** Before a group begins, the staff must be certain that a room or rooms will be available for all of the sessions. If this cannot be guaranteed beforehand, then those conducting the program may wish to delay initiating sessions until facilities are available.

3. **Recruit participants.** Various techniques that might be employed in this regard were detailed in the last section.

4. **Order information resources.** Make sure you have a sufficient quantity of group leader and client manuals. We have made a determined effort to insure that, outside of the two manuals that comprise Asthma Self-Management, those conducting the program will not require any additional materials.

5. **Obtain necessary equipment.** There are three types of items required for Asthma Self-Management. First, there is need of an overhead projector as transparencies are used in all of the sessions. An alternate strategy is to have the visuals made into slides. Second, name tags should be distributed and used, particularly during the initial sessions. Both staff and participants should go by their first name; this enhances the informal relationship that develops among participants and between participants and the staff. Finally, each participant should be furnished with a copy of the client manual prior to the first session. The patients should not be discouraged from taking notes during the sessions; however, note taking might impede discussion. It usually is unnecessary as most of the material is contained in the client manual.

6. **Convert the visual masters in each session into transparencies.** This can be done for all sessions before the program commences. By doing so, the staff is certain that they will be prepared for all seven sessions. You may also wish to use slides.

7. **Read all of the material in the leader and client manuals.** It is helpful to review prior to each session. No matter how many times you may have conducted Asthma Self-Management, you may need to refresh your memory with respect to what occurs during any given session.

8. **Decide on approaches and leading questions for discussion.** After the initial session, this is not much of a problem as you should anticipate many questions and be prepared to use them as the basis for discussion. However, by reviewing topics to be discussed during any one session, you can do a more thorough job of generating discussion.

9. **Assemble all supplies.** Before each session, assemble refreshments, snacks, name tags, etc. A supply of data information forms, such as the diary and report of an attack form, should also be made available.

SELECTING SUITABLE PATIENTS FOR ASTHMA SELF-MANAGEMENT PROGRAM

The following is a list of criteria that should be considered in recommending self-management training for asthma. The list is by no means exhaustive; it reflects major factors that you may wish to consider in conducting Asthma Self-Management.

1. **Patients must have a confirmed diagnosis of asthma.** Even though an individual can claim to be asthmatic, his or her asthma must be medically confirmed. Thus, it is necessary to screen anyone who volunteers for the program. It is likely that the quicker patients acquire and perform self-management skills following the confirmation of their asthma, the more they will benefit from self-management training. They have the opportunity to learn, from the outset, both appropriate attitudes and skills for the management of their disorder. The variable of asthma severity is not that significant in the self-management of asthma. Although some may argue that greater benefits accrue to those with severe asthma--and this is often the case--it is frequently the patient with mild asthma, who overuses hospital emergency rooms or does not take medication in a proper manner, that benefits most. Thus, anyone with asthma, no matter the severity of their disorder, can benefit from self-management training.

2. **Patients must have a personal physician.** Asthma Self-Management is designed to teach participants to become partners with their physicians in the treatment and management of asthma. It is, therefore, essential that participants have a personal physician in order for the program to be successful. It sometimes happens that patients will, as a result of self-management training, switch to another physician. It is not your role to encourage such a change; such an event takes place when participants themselves believe that they will receive better treatment if they go to a specialist such as an allergist and chest physician.

3. **Patients must be able to communicate and form a personal relationship with those conducting the group.** Kanfer and Schefft (1988) have noted this to be a necessary condition for any self-management program. This factor also holds true for patients involved with the self-management of their asthma. It has been our experience that, given the proper context for self-management training, almost every adult and child with asthma will communicate and form a personal relationship both with group leaders and other members of the group. For what is often the first time in their lives, they have the opportunity to share common experiences with others; thus, the problem usually is limiting communication within an atmosphere designed to foster such interactions.

4. **Patients must have the potential to perform the self-management skills required by Asthma Self-Management.** This has not proven to be a major consideration for participants of either Living With Asthma or Asthma Self-Management. The original program, Living With Asthma, was designed for use with asthmatic children and their families; thus, almost any youngster 6 years of age or older and his or her family can benefit from participation. Asthma Self-Management, on the other hand, is designed for use with asthmatic adults. Although there is individual variability in the value of the program to participants, the skills can be acquired and practiced by anyone of normal, even borderline intelligence. A major ingredient for success is the motivation of individual patients, not their ability to learn or to perform self-management skills for asthma.

5. **Patients must have the capacity to realistically choose the level of their activities and the settings in which they can function with some degree of autonomy.** Kanfer and Schefft (1988) have suggested this final criterion. It is most appropriate in the self-management of asthma because attacks warrant that a patient recognize his limits and seek medical attention. A role of a personal physician is to assist the patient in establishing these limits; a role of the patient is to be aware of personal limits and seek whatever medical attention is required to alleviate an attack. Patients must also be aware of settings, such as when they are in areas away from hospitals and clinics, where they will need to take greater responsibility for their asthma. Through self-management training they hopefully will know the skills they need to perform when medical attention is not immediately available, as well as the requisite steps to seek medical attention.

SAMPLE NEWS FACT SHEET

CONTACT:

    NAME: _____

    ADDRESS: _____

    PHONE NUMBER: _____

ASTHMA SELF-MANAGEMENT GROUPS

WHAT: Education groups for asthmatic patients that are designed to teach them how to better manage their disorder and to become partners with their physicians in the treatment and management of asthma.

FOR WHOM: Any adult with a diagnosis of asthma.

GIVEN BY: Your name and brief background of your sponsoring organization.

WHEN: Time and date of first meeting and how long the group will continue.

WHERE: Address and room for the class.

COST: None or a nominal fee to cover handout reproduction costs.

OTHER: Need for preregistration and confirmation of diagnosis of asthma before class. Phone number of the contact person or agency.

References

Kanfer, F. H. (1980). Self-management methods. In F. H. Kanfer & A. P. Goldstein (Eds.), Helping People Change (2nd ed.). New York: Pergamon Press.

Kanfer, F.H., & Schefft, B.K. (1988). Guiding the process of therapeutic change. Champaign, IL: Research Press.

Creer, T. L., Backial, M., Ullman, S., & Leung, P. (1986). Living With Asthma (1986). Part I: Manual for teaching parents the self-management of childhood asthma. Part 2: Manual for teaching children the self-management of asthma. (NIH Publication No. 86-2364: U. S. Department of Health & Human Services, Washington, D.C.)

SESSION ONE
PROGRAM OVERVIEW:
PRINCIPLES OF SELF-MANAGEMENT AND THE NATURE OF ASTHMA

GOALS
1. Introduce members of the group to each other.
2. Orient group members to the participatory nature of the sessions.
3. Outline the goals, targets, and skills which comprise self-management.
4. Provide an overview of Peak Flow Meter use.
5. Introduce the SOLVED Problems Exercise.
6. Describe the nature of asthma.
7. Describe the respiratory system.
8. Describe the diagnosis of asthma.
9. Compare asthma to other chronic obstructive lung disorder.
10. Discuss common myths associated with asthma.

EQUIPMENT
Name tags.
Paper and pencils for all participants.
Overhead projector.

SUPPLIES
Coffee, tea, snacks, or light lunch.

SESSION ONE OUTLINE

TOPIC/ ACTIVITY	REQUIRED MATERIAL	APPROXIMATE TIME ALLOWED
Welcome & introductions	Name tags	10 minutes
Nature of the group sessions		5 minutes
Self-management goals	Visual 1.01	5 minutes
Self-management targets	Visual 1.02	5 minutes
Self-management skills	Visual 1.03	5 minutes
Use of peak flow values	(Refer to Chapter 8, Client Manual) Visuals 1.04-1.05	15 minutes
SOLVED Problems exercise	Appendix & Chapter 7, Client Manual Visual 1.06	20 minutes
Describe asthma and the respiratory system	Visuals 1.07-1.16	30 minutes
Diagnosis of asthma and comparison to other chronic obstructive lung disorders	Visual 1.17, Schering Visualizer	10 minutes
Common asthma myths	Visual 1.18	5 minutes
Discussion		10 minutes
Homework	Asthma Medication Worksheet (Handout 1.1, Client Manual) Read Chapters 3 & 8	10 minutes

SESSION ONE TEACHING NOTES

Welcome and introductions

Introduce yourself and all participating staff members to the group. Share your special areas of training and experience that pertain to asthma and its management. Allow time for all group members to fill out their name tags and to introduce themselves.

Nature of the group sessions

Indicate that the group sessions will involve both lecture material and informal discussion and questions. The latter activities are the most important to the program. Participants should be encouraged to bring questions up as they arise or to save them for the end of the session when there will be time for discussion. As much as possible, allow the patients to answer each others' questions. The group leader's role is to respond to misinformation and to clarify any answers.

Self-Management Goals, Targets, and Skills

Goals. Before introducing the basic goals of self-management training, provide the group with an opportunity to discuss what goals they have set for themselves in coming to this program. Then introduce the group to three basic goals: (1) becoming an ally with one's physician in treating asthma; (2) limiting the impact of asthma on one's life; and (3) gaining more confidence in one's ability to manage asthma. (Visual 1.01)

Targets. Self-management targets fall into four areas: behaviors, environmental factors, psychological factors (thoughts and feelings), and somatic or bodily factors. A brief description of each of these areas will be sufficient. Try to convey to the group the interactive nature of these target areas. (See the background material on social learning theory and reciprocal determinism.) (See Visual 1.02)

Skills. The two principle skill areas in self-management are behaviors and thoughts. (Visual 1.03) Important behavioral skills include self-monitoring, medication compliance, etc. Problem solving is among the most important cognitive skills. Use the introduction of self-management skills as a bridge to the next two sections of Session One, a discussion and demonstration of the proper use of the peak flow meter (Visuals 1.04, 1.05) and use of the SOLVE problem solving exercise. (Visual 1.06)

Problem Solving: The SOLVED Problems Exercise

Provide everyone with a few examples of the completed SOLVED Problems worksheet. Along with self-monitoring, problem solving is a basic self-management skill used throughout the program. It is important that participants have a basic introduction to the exercise and can begin using it in the next two sessions. It is unlikely that there will be time for the group members to use the SOLVED Problems worksheet in this session. (Visual 1.06; Appendix & Chapter 7 in Client Manual)

Asthma and the Respiratory System

Asthma: A description. Present an overview of the basic characteristics of asthma including a brief description of: hyperreactivity of the airways, airway obstruction, and the reversible, intermittent, and variable characteristics of attacks. (See Visual 1.07)

The Respiratory System. Topics in this section include a description of respiration (gas exchange) and overview of the respiratory system anatomy (see Schering Visualizer, Visuals 1.08-1.16). It is important that group members understand the basic concepts and nature of respiration, rather than specific details of breathing. Extra information can be provided depending on the expertise of the group leader and the needs of a particular group.

Diagnosis of Asthma

Present general steps taken in diagnosing asthma. Through the use of Visuals (1.17), the diagnosis of asthma should be differentiated from the diagnosis of chronic bronchitis and emphysema. The latter disorders are known as chronic obstructive pulmonary diseases (COPD). Any fears that asthma necessarily leads to COPD must be allayed. Also, the steady and irrecoverable deterioration in lung function associated with COPD should be clearly distinguished from the reversible nature of obstructed breathing in asthma. (Visual 1.18).

Common Asthma Myths

Several common myths about asthma include: *Asthma is all in my head; My feelings cause my asthma; Everyone outgrows asthma; Asthma can be cured; Asthma will cause my breathing to get worse as I grow older;* and *People with asthma should not exercise.* After briefly discussing these myths, allow the group to generate any other "asthma facts" which they are unsure about.

Homework

Acquiring and performing self-management skills is stressed in this program by the development of a homework assignment assigned at the end of each session. These assignments are designed to highlight material covered in the current session or to sensitize the group members to important issues to be addressed in the next session.

Session One's homework requires that group members complete Handout 1.2, found in the Appendix of the Client Manual, entitled the Asthma Medication Worksheet. A Visual is provided to help introduce this form. Ask clients to also read Chapter 3 before the next session.

Discussion

Every session ends with an informal discussion of topics presented during that session. It is imperative that group leaders allow group members to answer questions among themselves. Group leaders can clarify or correct misinformation. Group participants are more likely to answer questions as the program progresses.

A Note About Visuals

There are two types of Visuals included in this manual, both of which are suitable for use as overheads. The first type are session outlines that can be used to structure the didactic presentations which consume most of the first few sessions. The second type of visual include diagrams, charts, or copies of forms used in the program (e.g., SOLVED Problems exercise). Individual group leaders should adapt the program to fit their style of presentation. Some leaders may prefer to use overheads to structure their presentations and/or to display the diagrams or charts, whereas others may wish to eliminate use of the overhead and to provide copies of the diagrams to each group member.

SESSION ONE BACKGROUND READING

USING PEAK EXPIRATORY FLOW RATE VALUES IN THE SELF-MANAGEMENT OF ASTHMA

Daily assessment of lung functions is important to individuals with asthma for at least two reasons. First, many asthmatics have inaccurate self-perceptions of airway obstruction (e.g., Rubenfield & Pain, 1976). The use of a portable peak flow meter can correct the problem by providing individuals with objective information about their degree of bronchoconstriction. Daily lung function assessment may also improve the ability of asthmatic patients to discriminate changes in airway obstruction (i.e., asthma severity), although empirical confirmation of this desired effect is often lacking (Higgs, Richardson, Lea, Lewis, & Laszlo, 1986; Sly, Landau, & Weymouth, 1985). Second, changes in daily lung function scores can be used to make decisions about implementing preventative self-management steps (e.g., drinking water, resting), changing one's medication regimen (e.g., increasing the dose of a medication), or seeking emergency medical treatment (Williams, 1982). Improving decision-making skills is a hallmark of effective self-management training (Creer & Reynolds, 1990).

Using lung function values in self-management decision making requires self-monitoring of asthma symptoms and lung function values for at least four weeks (see Harm, Kotses, & Creer, 1985). First, an individual must determine the probability of having an asthma attack in any given 12-hour period. This is known as the probability of asthma or the asthma episode base rate. Second, a cutoff value for the lung function score is determined. (Methods used to select the cutoff value are discussed in Harm et al. [1985].) The probability of an asthma episode increases when the lung function score is less than or equal to the cutoff value. Probability estimates based on peak expiratory flow rate (PEFR) data, collected twice daily by in-home use of the Mini-Wright Peak Flow Meter, have produced a three- to five-fold increase in the predictability of asthma episodes over base rate for asthmatic children (Harm et al., 1985; Taplin & Creer, 1978).

Clearly, lung function data and probability equations provide the technology for increasing the predictability of asthma episodes. However, research has yet to demonstrate that lung function data can be used by patients to improve self-management of their asthma. The only treatment study to date found that addition of asthma prediction training to self-management training yielded no additional improvement in the patients' ability to manage their asthma over the effects of the multicomponent self-management program alone (Marion, 1987).

Several technological and practical problems exist which may limit the effective use of lung function and probability data in asthma decision making and self-management. For example, when asthma episode base rates are very low or very high, there will be little or no improvement and, in some cases, there is a decrement in asthma episode prediction accuracy (Faust, 1986; Marion, 1987). This base rate problem was noted in at least two prediction studies (Harm et al., 1985; Marion, 1987). In addition, it is unclear whether patients will comply with self-management recommendations even in the face of increased probability of asthma; they may disregard lung function data as they do other symptom feedback. Making the prediction procedure as simple and clear as possible is likely to increase compliance. Finally, no study has demonstrated that the posterior probabilities will be useful during a follow-up period (Taplin & Creer, 1978). Although retrospective prediction of asthma may be improved substantially on the basis of lung function scores, accurate prospective prediction is far from certain.

Despite the technological limitations and clinical concerns noted, anecdotal observation of adults and children with asthma indicates that some patients make effective use of lung function data in the same way they make effective use of other self-monitored information such as daily changes in asthma symptoms (e.g., wheezing, fatigue). Thus, much work remains in the implementation and testing of asthma self-prediction methods.

SELF-MANAGEMENT AND SOCIAL LEARNING THEORY

Social learning theory organizes the therapeutic goals of the self-management of chronic illness into three areas: (1) self-control skills; (2) beliefs important to initiating and maintaining health behavior change are enhanced (e.g., efficacy and outcome expectancies); and (3) environmental conditions (including family and social networks). Training in self-control skills include cognitive and behavioral skills (e.g., self-monitoring or problem solving).

Sometimes, teaching a specific skill is sufficient to bring about important changes in health behavior and health status. For example, digital temperature biofeedback training produces long-term benefit in the treatment of Raynaud's disease (Freedman & Ianni, 1986). However, training in multiple self-management skills is more common in the management of chronic illness. Comprehensive self-management programs often include training in observational and self-monitoring skills, problem-solving and decision-making skills, and specific self-control behaviors (e.g., avoiding asthma triggers).

Beliefs that enhance the effective performance of self-management skills include expectations of success or personal efficacy. Self-efficacy is defined as the belief that one can successfully perform specific behaviors such as self-monitoring or other self-management behaviors (Bandura, 1977; 1982; 1984). The strength of an individuals' expectations for successful performance determine how much effort they will put forth and how long they will persist in their coping efforts (Bandura, 1977; 1980). Outcome expectancies, the belief that a specific behavior will lead to a desired outcome (i.e., rewards), is also thought to affect people's performance of self-management or coping behavior (Bandura, 1984; Godding & Glasgow, 1985). Regarding asthma self-management, it is easy to see how these two types of beliefs can influence the performance of self-management behavior. For example, the performance of peak expiratory flow rate (PEFR) self-monitoring is dependent on the belief that one can accurately perform the PEFR maneuver (self-efficacy), and that the monitoring, recording, and charting of PEFR will result in improved asthma management as seen by fewer asthma episodes of lesser severity (outcome expectancies).

The final component of Bandura's social learning model involves the client's management of the environment--i.e., developing environmental conditions that support the change in health behavior and improved health status. This can include social skills training to improve the use of support systems or structuring the environment so that healthy behaviors will be followed (e.g., posting medication reminders around the home).

Other theorists have extended the social learning model to include a physiological (somatic) dimension (Thoresen & Kirmil-Gray, 1983). Somatic variables important in the self-management of asthma include blood levels of theophylline-based medications (e.g., Stine, Marcus, & Parvin, 1987), and immunological factors that mediate the hypersecretion of mucous and hyperactivity of the smooth muscles in the lung (Ingram, 1987). Peak expiratory flow is an important somatic variable which asthmatics can assess at home.

Although the possible interactions of the dimensions of social learning theory create a complicated model, it is a useful heuristic for thinking about assessment and intervention in individual cases. (See Tobin, Reynolds, Holroyd, & Creer [1986] for a review of social learning theory and self-management.)

TIPS FOR EXERCISING

There are a number of tips for exercising that should be considered by the patient with asthma (Table 1:1).

TABLE 1:1. TIPS FOR EXERCISING FOR THE PATIENT WITH ASTHMA

Exercise and be physically fit

Discuss exercise options with physician

Discuss premedication needs with physician

Discuss whether you need to keep a
  bronchodilator present during exercise

Warm up with light exercise

In cold or dry weather, wear a mask over
  nose and mouth

Cool down with light exercise

If you still experience exercise-induced asthma:

  1. Switch to a different exercise activity

  2. Review need for asthma medications with
     physician

Know your limits for exercising

Motivate yourself to exercise regularly

These include:

1.   It is important that the patient with asthma exercise and remain physically fit. As with their non-asthmatic peers, the better condition the patient is in, the less debilitating will be their disorder. Furthermore, if he or she ever experiences a severe attack, the question of survival could hinge on the physical fitness of the individual.

2. Before exercising, the patient should discuss possible options with his or her physician. The latter may not only recommend how much exercise should be obtained, but what would be the best activity for the patient. Many physicians believe that swimming, particularly in a heated pool, is the optimal type of exercise for asthmatic patients; others, however, believe that if the patient is careful, he or she can engage in almost any type of exercise.

3. If needed, the physician may prescribe that the patient take a medication 15 to 30 minutes prior to exercising. The most common types of medications used to prevent exercise-induced asthma are cromolyn sodium, such as Intal, or albuterol, usually Proventil and Ventolin.

4. The asthmatic patient should warm up with light exercise before engaging in a more vigorous workout. As with their non-asthmatic peers, the patient with asthma should begin with short workouts and gradually increase the amount of time engaged in such activity.

5. In cold or dry weather, patients may wish to wear a mask over their mouth and nose. This permits the air to be heated and moisturized before progressing too far down into the bronchial tubes. By becoming properly heated and moisturized, there is less of a likelihood that the cold or dry air can bring on an asthma flare-up.

6. As in all exercise, the asthmatic patient should cool down with light exercise. This will permit his or her breathing to adjust to normal levels.

7. The asthmatic patient may wish to keep a bronchodilator on hand if exercise is a trigger of his or her attacks. With the beginning of wheezing or tightness of the chest, the patient may wish to use self-management exercises such as relaxing and drinking warm or tepid liquids. If this does not seem to reverse the breathing impediment, then the patient will wish to inhale a dose from the bronchodilator.

8. If the patient still experiences exercise-induced asthma, he or she may consider two strategies: First, he or she may wish to try a different form of exercise. Instead of performing an activity that requires constant running, such as basketball, the patient may wish to switch to an exercise such as tennis. Second, the patient may wish to contact his or her physician to determine whether the patient needs to change medications to prevent exercise-induced asthma.

9. The patient with asthma is in the best position to decide how much exercise is enough at any given time. Although physicians can provide advice and prescribe medications to be taken to prevent attacks, it is up to the patient to know his or her limits during any given workout. This fact is not lost upon professional athletes who, upon experiencing the initial signs of an attack, will take themselves out of the game, exercise whatever action is necessary to control the episode, and then resume whatever activity they were performing.

10. Finally, asthmatic patients must, like everyone else, realize that they must motivate themselves to exercise regularly. Having asthma is not a valid excuse for failing to keep oneself in good physical condition; being in shape, on the other hand, can bring considerable rewards through health and well-being to the patient with asthma.

SEVEN REASONS WHY SELF-MANAGEMENT IS SIGNIFICANT IN THE CONTROL OF ASTHMA

Kanfer and Schefft (1988) have stated that there are seven reasons why self-management is often selected to change behavior (Table 1:2).

TABLE 1:2. SEVEN REASONS WHY SELF-MANAGEMENT IS SIGNIFICANT

According to Kanfer & Schefft (1988):

1. Perceived control increases motivation

2. Pursuing and attaining goals act as a source of motivation

3. Self-management lowers noncompliance

4. Perception of control enhances self-efficacy

5. Self-attributions following self-management reinforce independent actions

6. Self-management is ethically and socially valued more than passive treatment

7. Self-management facilitates generalization of treatment effects

---

These factors are significant in the self-management of asthma in the following ways:

1. **Perceived control increases motivation.** A patient's participation in setting goals and cooperating in his asthma treatment leads to a greater investment of energy, makes the treatment goals more attractive, and yields greater effort towards their achievement.

2. **Pursuing and attaining goals, set in cooperation with their physician, acts as a source of motivation.** The process of managing one's own behavior is, in itself, challenging and rewarding . Patients are more apt to perform self-management skills to prove to themselves and their physicians that they can do them.

3. **Self-management lowers noncompliance.** Patients who feel themselves partners with their physicians in the treatment of asthma can use their knowledge and skills in discussing treatment strategies. They are more likely to comply with whatever regimens are developed and, conversely, less likely to sabotage treatment.

4. **Perception of control enhances self-efficacy.** The ability to participate in therapeutic decisions tends to enhance patients' self-efficacy or beliefs about their own abilities.

5. **Self-attributions following self-management reinforce independent actions.** When patients perceive themselves as the source of progress made in the control of their asthma, their increased self-confidence helps them take further steps in asthma management, and to show a greater willingness to autonomously make initial treatment steps.

6. **Self-management is ethically and socially-valued more than passive treatment.** Patient participation reduces the introduction of distracting issues of value choices and patient rights that can arise in medical treatment.

7. **Self-management facilitates generalization of treatment effects.** When patients learn to regulate their own actions, their dependence upon external direction and cues is decreased. Maintenance of gains made by patients can be supported by self-generated cues and reinforcement.

SIX THINK RULES ABOUT THE SELF-MANAGEMENT OF ASTHMA

Kanfer and Schefft (1988) have proposed six think rules as important elements in changing behavior. The significance of these for you are as follows:

1. **Think Behavior.** Assist the patient to redefine problems about asthma in behavioral terms.

2. **Think Solution.** Teach the patient to continually ask, "What is the most I can do to improve my asthma?"

3. **Think Positive.** Teach the patient to identify personal strengths and the positive aspects of any event or change effort.

4. **Think Small Steps.** Have the patient initially set limited goals to enhance the likelihood of success and to permit continuing reappraisal.

5. **Think Flexible.** Teach the patient to develop alternatives and back-up plans and to be prepared for the unexpected.

6. **Think Future.** Teach the patient to focus on the future and encourage rehearsal and planning.

References

Bandura, A. (1977). Self-efficacy: Toward a unifying theory of behavior change. Psychological Review, 84, 191-215.

Bandura, A. (1982). Self-efficacy in human agency. American Psychologist, 37, 122-147.

Bandura, A. (1984). Recycling misconceptions of perceived self-efficacy. Cognitive Therapy and Research, 8, 231-255.

Creer, T. L., & Reynolds, R. V. (1990). Asthma. In A. M. Gross & R. S. Drabman (Eds.), Handbook of clinical behavioral pediatrics. New York: Plenum Press.

Faust, D. (1986). Research on human judgment and its application to clinical practice. Professional Psychology: Research and Practice, 17, 420-430.

Freedman, R. R., & Ianni, P. (1986). Raynaud's disease. In K. A. Holroyd & T. L. Creer (Eds.), Self-management of chronic disease. Handbook of clinical interventions and research. Orlando, FL: Academic Press.

Godding, P. R., & Glasgow, R. E. (1985). Self-efficacy and outcome expectations as predictors of controlled smoking status. Cognitive Therapy and Research, 9, 583-590.

Harm, D. L., Kotses, H., & Creer, T. L. (1985). Improving the ability of peak expiratory flow rates to predict asthma. Journal of Allergy and Clinical Immunology, 76, 688-694.

Higgs, C. M. B., Richardson, R. B., Lea, D. A., Lewis, G. T. R., & Laszlo, G. (1986). Influence of knowledge of peak flow on self assessment of asthma: Studies with a coded peak flow meter. Thorax, 41, 671-675.

Ingram, R. H. (1987). Research need: Unresolved questions about the etiology of asthma. Chest, 91, 1935-1945.

Kanfer, F. H., & Schefft, B. K. (1988). Guiding the process of therapeutic change. Champaign, IL: Research Press.

Marion, R. J. (1987). Teaching children to predict asthma using an in-home pulmometer. Unpublished doctoral dissertation, Ohio University, Athens, Ohio.

Rubinfeld, A. R., & Pain, M. C. (1976). Perception of asthma. Lancet, 1, 882-884.

Sly, P. D., Landau, L. I., & Weymouth, R. (1985). Home recording of peak expiratory flow rates and perception of asthma. American Journal of Diseases in Children, 139, 479-482.

Stine, R. J., Marcus, R. H., & Parvin, C. A. (1987). Clinical predictors of theophylline blood levels in asthmatic patients. Annals of Emergency Medicine, 16, 18-24.

Taplin, P. S., & Creer, T. L. (1978). A procedure for using peak expiratory flow rate data to increase the predictability of asthma episodes. Journal of Asthma Research, 16, 15-19.

Thoresen, C. E., & Kirmil-Gray, K. (1983). Self-management psychology and the treatment of childhood asthma. Journal of Allergy and Clinical Immunology, 72, 596-606.

Tobin, D. L., Reynolds, R. V., Holroyd, K. A., & Creer, T. L. (1986). Self-management and social learning theory. In K. A. Holroyd & T. L. Creer (Eds.), Self-management of chronic disease Handbook of clinical interventions and research. Orlando, FL: Academic Press.

Williams, M. H., Jr. (1982). Expiratory flow rates: Their role in asthma therapy. Hospital Practice, 17, 95-110.

SELF-MANAGEMENT GOALS
VISUAL 1.01

BECOME AN ALLY WITH YOUR PHYSICIAN

LIMIT THE IMPACT OF ASTHMA ON YOUR LIFE

GAIN MORE CONFIDENCE IN YOUR ABILITY TO MANAGE YOUR ASTHMA FLAREUPS AND ATTACKS

SELF-MANAGEMENT TARGETS
VISUAL 1.02

BEHAVIORS
Exercise

Medication noncompliance

ENVIRONMENT
Allergens

Irritants

Pharmaceuticals (e.g., aspirin)

PSYCHOLOGICAL VARIABLES
Emotional responses

Outcome expectancies

Self-efficacy

SOMATIC VARIABLES
Stress level

Respiratory infections

<u>SELF-MANAGEMENT SKILLS</u>
VISUAL 1.03

BEHAVIORS
Self-monitoring

Medication compliance

Avoiding triggers

Active use of health care

Attack Management Behaviors
1. Rest and relax.
2. Drink liquids.
3. Take medications as prescribed.
4. Contact family or friends if necessary.

COGNITIVE SKILLS
Self-statements

Problem solving/decision making

PROPER USE OF A PEAK FLOW METER
VISUAL 1.04

1. Be sure that any food or gum is out of your mouth.

2. Hold the meter parallel to the ground.

3. Be sure that the pointer is as close to your lips as it can go.

4. Inhale as much air as you can.

5. Put your mouth completely over the mouth-piece, with your lips tight around it and your tongue out of the way.

6. Blow out as hard and as fast as you can.

7. Still keeping the meter parallel to the ground, check to see where the pointer is now.

8. Reset the pointer as close to your lips as possible and blow again, following the same instructions as before.

9. Again, reset the pointer to the beginning and blow.

10. Write down on your weekly asthma diary the <u>highest</u> of your three blows.

11. Be sure to record your peak flow <u>every</u> day, once in the morning and again in the evening.

<u>USE OF PEAK FLOW VALUES IN ASTHMA SELF-MANAGEMENT</u>

VISUAL 1.05

1. Confirm an asthma attack.

2. Compare the sensations of asthma against a peak flow value.

3. Predict the likelihood of an asthma attack during a particular period of time.

4. Determine if an attack has worsened and whether you need to initiate further treatment.

SOLVED PROBLEMS EXERCISE
VISUAL 1.06

1. **S**TATE THE PROBLEM

2. **O**UTLINE THE PROBLEM

3. **L**IST POSSIBLE SOLUTIONS

4. **V**IEW POSSIBLE CONSEQUENCES

5. **E**XECUTE YOUR SOLUTIONS

6. **D**ETERMINE SOLUTION'S EFFECTIVENESS

ASTHMA: A DESCRIPTION
VISUAL 1.07

HYPERRRESPONSIVE AIRWAYS
Allergens
Irritants
Exercise
Respiratory Infections
Aspirin and related substances
Emotional responses

AIRWAY OBSTRUCTION
REVERSIBILITY

INTERMITTENT NATURE

VARIABILITY

THE RESPIRATORY SYSTEM AND ASTHMA

VISUAL 1.08

RESPIRATION: O_2 AND CO_2 EXCHANGE

ANATOMY OF THE RESPIRATORY SYSTEM	(Visual 1.09)
OXYGEN EXCHANGE IN THE ALVEOLI	(Visual 1.10)
MUSCLES OF BREATHING	(Visual 1.11)
AIR IS CLEANED	(Visual 1.12)
AIR IS MOISTURIZED AND WARMED	(Visual 1.13)
AIRFLOW AND THE MUSCLES SURROUNDING THE AIRWAYS	(Visual 1.14)
BREATHING AWARENESS	
WHAT HAPPENS DURING AN ASTHMA ATTACK	(Visual 1.15)
TRAPPED AIR	(Visual 1.16)

1. NORMAL **LUNGS**

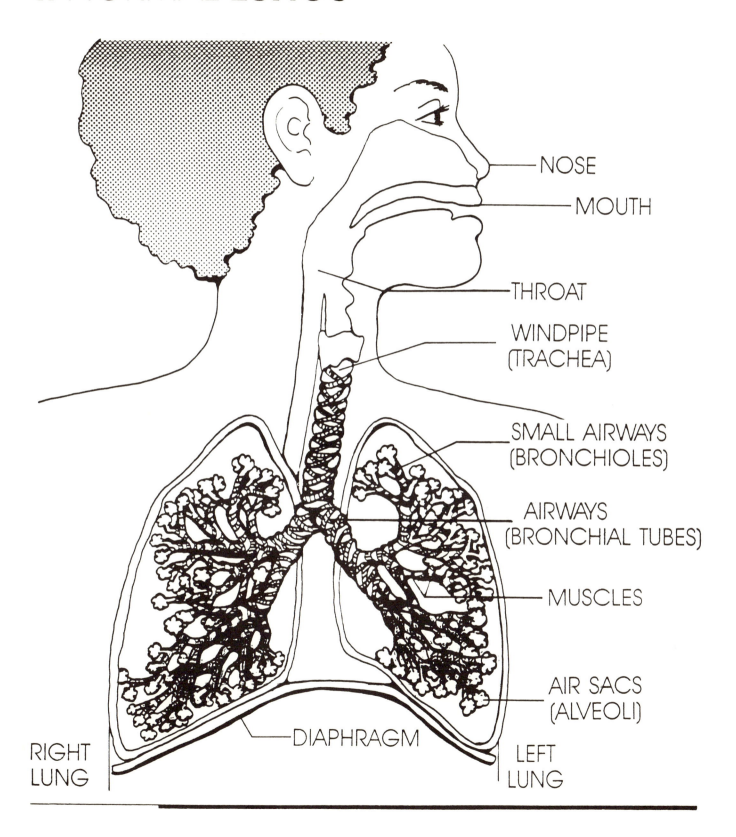

NOSE

MOUTH

THROAT

WINDPIPE
(TRACHEA)

SMALL AIRWAYS
(BRONCHIOLES)

AIRWAYS
(BRONCHIAL TUBES)

MUSCLES

AIR SACS
(ALVEOLI)

DIAPHRAGM

RIGHT
LUNG

LEFT
LUNG

2. OXYGEN EXCHANGE IN THE AIR SACS

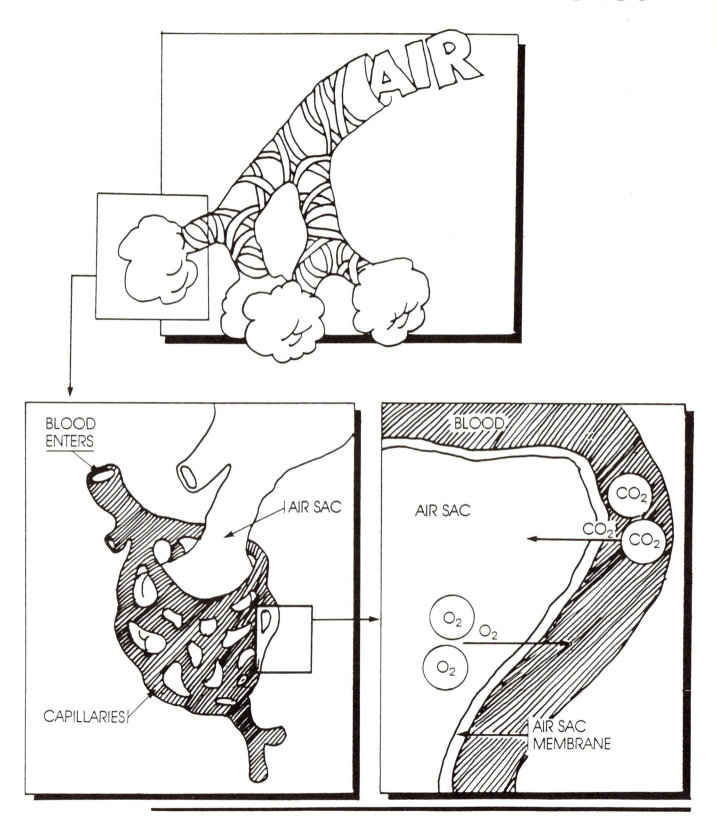

3. MUSCLES OF BREATHING

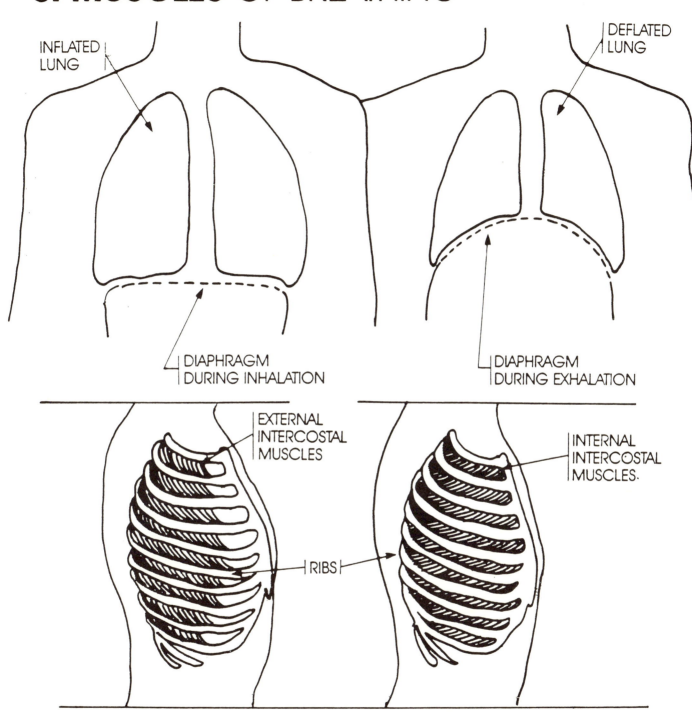

INFLATED LUNG

DEFLATED LUNG

DIAPHRAGM DURING INHALATION

DIAPHRAGM DURING EXHALATION

EXTERNAL INTERCOSTAL MUSCLES

INTERNAL INTERCOSTAL MUSCLES.

RIBS

CHEST WALL MUSCLES—EXTERNAL AND INTERNAL INTERCOSTAL MUSCLES
SIDE VIEW

4. AIR IS **CLEANED**

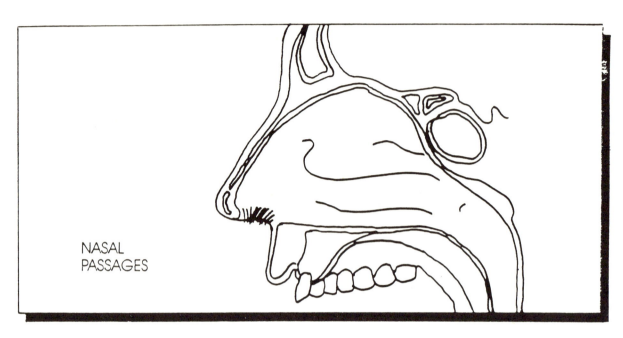

NASAL
PASSAGES

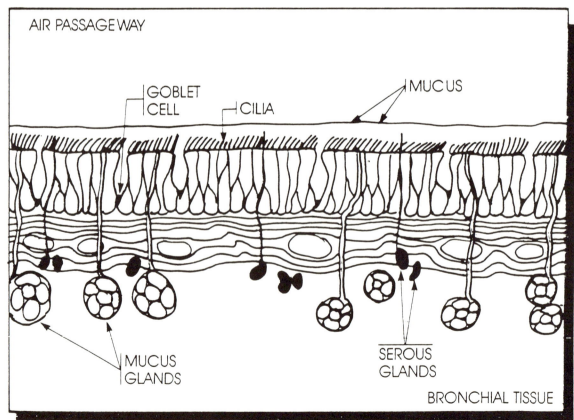

AIR PASSAGEWAY

GOBLET
CELL

CILIA

MUCUS

MUCUS
GLANDS

SEROUS
GLANDS

BRONCHIAL TISSUE

5. AIR IS **MOISTURIZED**

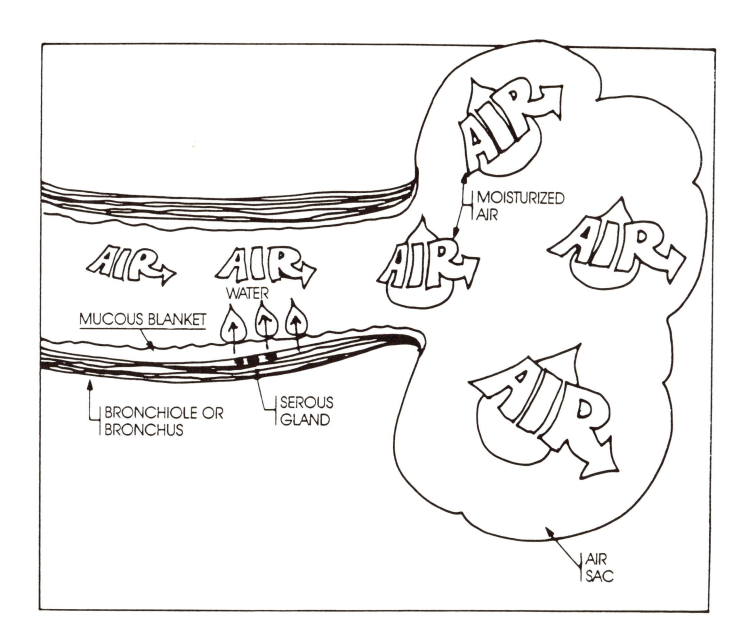

6. MUSCLES SURROUNDING AIRWAYS

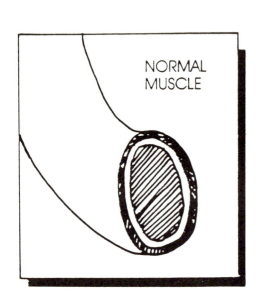

NORMAL MUSCLE

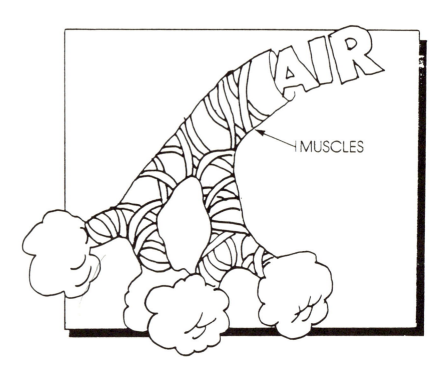

AIR

MUSCLES

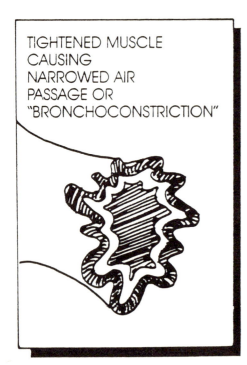

TIGHTENED MUSCLE CAUSING NARROWED AIR PASSAGE OR "BRONCHOCONSTRICTION"

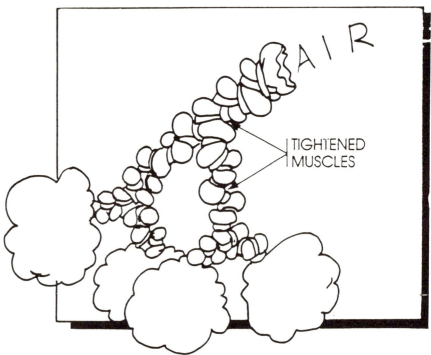

AIR

TIGHTENED MUSCLES

7. WHAT HAPPENS DURING AN ASTHMA ATTACK

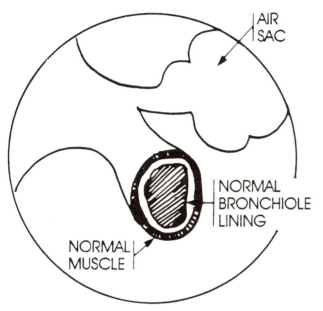

NORMAL INTERIOR OF BRONCHIOLE

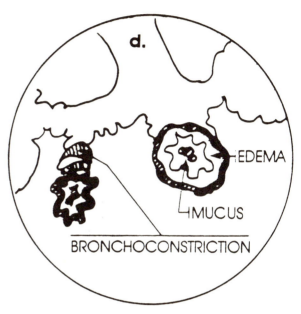

INTERIOR OF BRONCHIOLE
DURING AN ASTHMA ATTACK

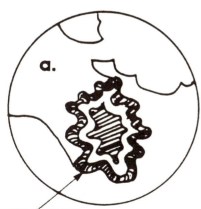

TIGHTENED
MUSCLE CAUSING
NARROWED AIR
PASSAGE OR
"BRONCHOCONSTRICTION"

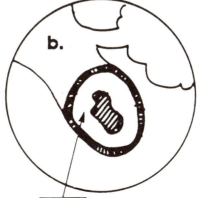

EDEMA
(SWELLING OF THE
LINING OF THE
BRONCHIAL TUBE)

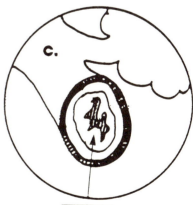

MUCUS
SECRETION

8. AIR **TRAPPING** AND BUILD-UP OF CO_2 IN AIR SACS

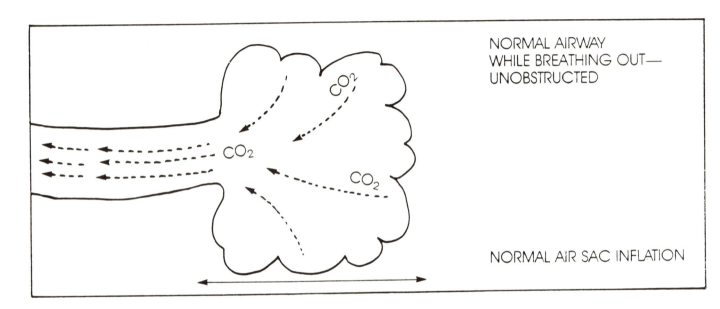

NORMAL AIRWAY
WHILE BREATHING OUT—
UNOBSTRUCTED

NORMAL AIR SAC INFLATION

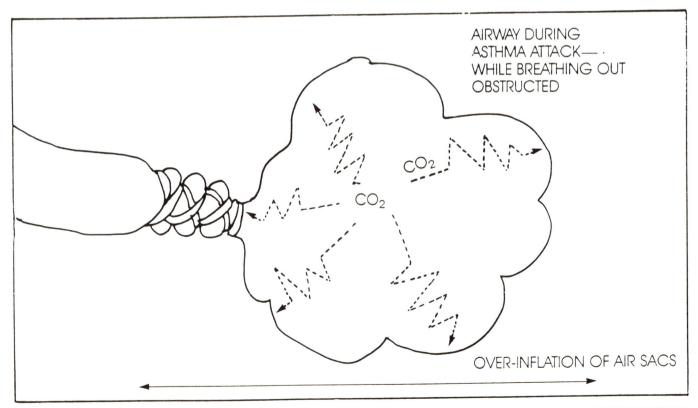

AIRWAY DURING
ASTHMA ATTACK—
WHILE BREATHING OUT
OBSTRUCTED

OVER-INFLATION OF AIR SACS

THE DIAGNOSIS OF ASTHMA
VISUAL 1.17

HISTORY AND PHYSICAL

Symptoms: cough, wheeze, shortness of
breath

Triggers

Skin testing

Oral challenge

LUNG FUNCTION TESTS

Airway obstruction

20% or greater decrease in FEV_1 when

inhaling chemicals known to produce
bronchoconstriction

Airway hyperresponsiveness

Exercise challenge

Bronchial challenge

Response to treatment

15% or greater improvement in FEV_1

when a bronchodilator is inhaled

OTHER RESPIRATORY DISORDERS

EMPHYSEMA

Enlargement of small airspaces

Lost elasticity

CHRONIC BRONCHITIS

Excess mucus production

COMMON ASTHMA MYTHS
VISUAL 1.18

ASTHMA IS IN THE HEAD

FEELINGS CAUSE ASTHMA

EVERYONE OUTGROWS ASTHMA

ASTHMA CAN BE CURED

ASTHMA CAUSES BREATHING TO GET PROGRESSIVELY WORSE

INDIVIDUALS WITH ASTHMA SHOULD NOT EXERCISE

SESSION TWO
ASTHMA MEDICATIONS

GOALS
1. Discuss common asthma medications and their use.
2. Review self-management issues related to the use of asthma medications.
3. Discuss problems with medication side effects and medication compliance

EQUIPMENT
Name tags.

Paper and pencils for all participants.

UPSC asthma medication information handouts (optional).

Overhead projector or slide projector.

Blackboard or grease pen and blank sheets for overhead.

SUPPLIES
Coffee, tea, snacks, or light lunch.

SESSION TWO OUTLINE

TOPIC/ ACTIVITY	REQUIRED MATERIAL	APPROXIMATE TIME ALLOWED
Welcome & salutations	Name tags	5 minutes
Questions about prior sessions and readings		10 minutes
Overview of asthma medications	Blackboard Asthma Medication Worksheet (Handout 1.1, Client Manual) Asthma Drug Names (Chapter 3, Client Manual) Visuals 2.1-2.6	45 minutes
Immunotherapy	Visual 2.7	10 minutes
Medication compliance	Asthma Medication Worksheet (Handout 1.1, Client Manual)	20 minutes
Homework	Early Warning Signs Worksheet (Handout 2.1, Client Manual) Read Chapter 4	10 minutes

SESSION TWO TEACHING NOTES

Welcome and Salutations

Put out the name tags. Allow time for group small talk prior to getting into the session material.

Questions About Prior Sessions/Readings

Allow the group time to ask questions about material covered in Session I.

Overview of Asthma Medications

Session 2 provides participants with a thorough overview of basic information about asthma drugs. The leader may present as much or as little information as the group's needs and attention allow. Integral to the session is a guest physician, pharmacist, or other health care professional to answer specific questions about medications. The guest professional may also wish to present the basic information about asthma drugs; be certain to know his or her preferences beforehand.

Some of the information may be conveyed through a discussion in which the leader asks questions of the group and corrects any misunderstandings they may have. In addition to basic information, participants should come to understand a number of concepts related to self-management:

1. The importance of knowing the exact names of the asthma medicines that are prescribed and the times they should be taken.

2. The concept of therapeutic level.

3. The importance of taking daily asthma medicines on time.

4. Knowledge of the side effects of asthma medicines.

5. Realizing that side effects of the medications can affect one's behavior and physical condition.

6. Knowing that medications can be taken before exercise or before exposure to allergens to prevent attacks, allowing individuals to participate in more activities.

7. Being aware of the pros and cons of using nebulized bronchodilators.

8. Finding ways to avoid overuse of nebulized bronchodilators:

   a. Not carrying the nebulizer

   b. Informing individuals about the bronchoconstriction that can occur if the inhaled bronchodilator is overused.

   c. Helping participants not to panic during an attack so he/she will avoid the urgency to use and reuse the nebulized medication.

These points may be stressed during the discussions in response to participants' comments.

Not everyone uses nebulized bronchodilators (nebs, for short); thus, they are not an issue for patients that do use them. If nebs are not a problem with the group, then a discussion of the topic may be omitted or treated only briefly.

A number of handouts are available. These include helpful facts and hints about asthma medicines, a guidesheet for asking the family physician questions about the medications, and common questions and answers about asthma medicines. These may be distributed as information sheets or built into session activities with class interactions engineered by the group leader.

Session Structure

Ask everyone to list the asthma medications they are currently taking, and to indicate what dose is prescribed and how often it is taken. Write the name of the medicines on the overhead or blackboard as they are mentioned. As you continue, list only those medications that have not been mentioned. If a previously cited brand name is given, put a small check next to the name each time it is noted. This will provide a picture of which drugs are most commonly used by participants.

As you write the brand names on the board, leave space for five categories; place together all the names corresponding to the following categories: (1) xanthines; (2) adrenergic bronchodilators; (3) cromolyn sodium; (4) anticholinergic bronchodilators; and (5) steroids. Consult the Asthma Drug Names chart included in Chapter 3 of the client manual. For adrenergics and steroids, you can subdivide each list into two parts for both oral and inhaled forms. Regular use of injected forms of medications is unlikely to be reported.

This exercise is designed to sensitize group members to differences in medication regimens.

Allow discussion of the similarities and differences in asthma medication regimens. Next, using Visuals 2.1-2.5, review the use of each class of asthma medication. Promote discussion of side effects as each class of medications is presented, and encourage participants to draw on their Asthma Medication Worksheet.

Chapter 3 in the client manual provides a good overview of this material. In addition, some background reading is provided in this manual. Refer participants to the Asthma Drug Names chart in their materials for this session.

Medication Compliance

Ask for a show of hands for participants who took a medication late or missed a dose altogether during this past week. Make a list of circumstances or factors that encouraged noncompliance with medications. Facilitate discussion of medication noncompliance by encouraging better compliance, yet openly acknowledging the difficulties and roadblocks to good compliance. Only through an awareness and acceptance of the environmental and personal factors that impede compliance can participants improve their record in this area.

Homework

Teach the clients how to complete the Early Warning Signs Worksheet, Handout 2.1. There are two sections to this handout with one part completed by the client and the other completed by a significant other. Also, ask that Chapter 4 be read prior to the next session.

SESSION TWO BACKGROUND READING

THEOPHYLLINE

Methylxanthines, administered in the form of a strong coffee, were used as a remedy for asthma in the middle of the 19th century. Beginning in the 1930s, theophylline was used for the treatment of asthma. In addition to its use as a medication for the treatment of asthma, theophylline is frequently prescribed as a prophylactic agent in the treatment of chronic asthma. Increased knowledge of the pharmacokinetics and pharmacodynamics of theophylline, and the introduction of sustained-release dosage forms have made theophylline the most frequently prescribed antiasthmatic medication in the United States.

MECHANISMS OF ACTION

It Is Known That Theophylline:

1. Indirectly inhibits the release of mediators from the mast cells. This would include: (a) altering the intracellular disposition of the calcium in the tracheal smooth muscle that is available for muscle contraction; and (b) antagonizing adenosine, a mediator that enhances degranulation of the mast cells, thus producing bronchoconstriction.

2. Is a potent smooth muscle relaxant; and,

3. Is possibly an anti-inflammatory agent.

THERAPEUTIC RANGE

The minimal effective concentration of theophylline is thought to be 10 mcg/ml. The upper limit of 20 mcg/ml is set in an attempt to minimize the risk of toxicity. The lower limit is less definitive and should be based on the individual patient's clinical response.

Three Factors Affect Fluctuations in Serum Theophylline Concentrations:

1. PATIENT SPECIFIC: The rate of elimination can vary by more than twofold in any population. Those with rapid elimination will likely have larger fluctuations in serum theophylline concentrations, whereas those with slow elimination tend to have smaller fluctuations.

2. PRODUCT SELECTION: There are more than two dozen sustained release theophylline products available for use in the U.S. Many of these are sufficiently distinct that they should not be considered therapeutically interchangeable. Rate and extent of absorption of a particular product will affect fluctuations in serum theophylline concentrations that are observed.

3. DOSAGE INTERVAL: This interval is selected by the patient's physician. Theoretically, a shorter dosage interval will provide less fluctuation in serum theophylline concentrations. However, patient acceptance and compliance may be potentially enhanced by selecting less frequent dosage intervals. Selecting a dosage regimen with sustained release theophylline should be tailored to meet the specific needs of the individual patient.

TABLE 2:1. SOME CAUSES OF LOWER OR HIGHER SERUM THEOPHYLLINE CONCENTRATIONS

Lower serum theophylline concentrations than expected may be due to:

1. Dose, sampling time, and compliance;

2. Age (1-16 years);

3. Use of drugs including phenobarbital, phenytoins, carbamazepine (tegretol) aminoglutethimide, and marijuana;

4. Dietary factors, such as a change from low protein-high carbohydrate to high protein-low carbohydrate, or inclusion of a large amount of charcoal-broiled foods, can also increase metabolism; and

5. Tobacco.

Higher serum theophylline concentrations than expected may be due to:

1. Overcompliance or overuse of medications;

2. Interaction with other medications, such as intravenous isoproternol, TAO or erythromycin antibodies, oral contraceptives, allopurinol (zyloprim, cimetidine, Tagamet), may produce higher serum theophylline levels;

3. Diseases that directly or indirectly influence liver function (specifically cirrhosis), congestive heart failure, COPD, cor pulmonale, or prolonged fever;

4. Influenza A vaccine;

5. Older age (>50 years);

6. Obesity; and

7. High-carbohydrate, low-protein diets.

TABLE 2:2. COMMON SIDE EFFECTS OF THEOPHYLLINE

1. Nausea;

2. Stomach cramps;

3. Stomach acidity and gastric problems;

4. Vomiting;

5. Diarrhea;

6. Headache;

7. Restlessness;

8. Tremor and shakiness;

9. Insomnia; and

10. Hyper-like behaviors.

THEOPHYLLINE LEVELS

PEAK LEVEL: Indicates whether there is too much theophylline in the patient's bloodstream, as well as whether the theophylline dose is sufficient.

THERAPEUTIC LEVEL: The lowest amount of theophylline required by the patient to control his or her asthma with minimal side effects.

TROUGH LEVEL: Indicates whether there is rapid theophylline breakdown, which could result in symptoms of asthma occurring sooner than anticipated.

TABLE 2:3.   BETA-AGONISTS/ADRENERGIC BRONCHODILATORS

Sympathomimetic drugs have been used since antiquity. For more than 5,000 years, the Chinese used Ma Muang, derived from a plant. Ephedrine was described in 1926; epinephrine was first discussed in 1900. It became a medication when the chemical adrenalin was discovered; this proved to be identical to epinephrine.

ADVANTAGES OF BETA-AGONISTS

1. Initial medication of choice for out-of-control asthma;

2. Helps keep airways open, sometimes at cost of side-effects; and

3. As they are dispensed via an inhaler, beta-agonists act directly on the airways.

SIDE EFFECTS OF SYMPATHOMIMETIC BRONCHODILATORS

Cardiovascular: Tachycardia, palpitations, arrhythmias, changes in blood pressure, angina, myocardial necrosis, vasoconstriction or vasodilation.

Nervous System: Agitation, anxiety, tremulousness, insomnia, faintness, dizziness, nervousness, and headache.

Genitourinary: Urinary retention (mainly in men with prostatic hypertrophy).

Ophthalmic: Glaucoma.

Metabolic: Hyperglycemia, and hyperthyroidism.

Gastrointestinal: Dry mouth, gagging, nausea, and vomiting.

Respiratory: Tracheal irritation, bronchial irritation, bronchospasm, cough, and dyspnea.

Pregnancy: Inhibition of premature labor.

Blood gases: Decrease in PaO_2.

Interaction with other drugs: Monoamine oxidase inhibitors, general anesthetics, hypotensive agents, pressor agents, thyroid hormone, insulin, oral hypoglycemic agents.

Other: Tachyphylaxis, paradoxic response (bronchospasm).

TABLE 2:4. EFFECTS OF ADRENORECEPTOR SIMULATION IN HUMANS

Alpha

1. Decreased adrenal cyclase activity;

2. Constriction of smooth muscle of veins, arteries;

3. Constriction of gastrointestinal, urinary bladder, trigone sphincters;

4. Enhanced histamine release;

5. Eosinophilia, platelet aggregation;

6. Contraction of pilomotor muscles;

7. Hepatic glycogenolysis, glucagon release;

8. Inhibition of insulin release; and

9. Inhibition of lipolysis.

Beta

1. Increased adrenyl cyclase activity;

2. Cardiac stimulation: inotropic, chronotropic;

3. Vasodilation, bronchodilation;

4. Uterine relaxation;

5. Bladder relaxation;

6. Eosinophenia, lymphopenia, granulocytosis;

7. Decreased lysosomal enzyme release;

8. Decreased lymphokine production;

9. Inhibition of histamine release;

10. Skeletal muscle tremor;

11. Muscle glycogenolysis;

12. Insulin release;

13. Gluconeogenesis; and,

14. Lipolysis.

CROMOLYN SODIUM

The discovery of cromolyn sodium evolved from an initial interest in a drug made from the seeds of a Mediterranean plant. While the drug had bronchodilator effects, it also produced gastrointestinal side-effects. This was remedied in 1965 with the synthesis of the white, odorless cromolyn sodium.

MODES OF ACTION

Three potential modes of action have been postulated:

1. Prevention of mast cell mediator release;

2. Modulation of reflex-induced bronchoconstriction under certain conditions; and,

3. Reduction in selected patients of nonspecific bronchial hyperactivity.

ADVANTAGES OF CROMOLYN SODIUM

1. Its broad therapeutic index and low risk-to-benefit ratio. Cromolyn exhibits a remarkably low order of acute toxicity, and has no described neoplastic or teratogenic properties.

2. Its actions are limited primarily to the lung, thereby minimizing the effect of treatment on other organ systems.

3. It is an effective preventive medication for: (a) exercise-induced asthma; (b) cold-air-induced asthma; and, (c) avoiding attacks that may be precipitated by anticipated allergens.

IT MUST BE EMPHASIZED THAT CROMOLYN SODIUM PREVENTS ATTACKS. IT IS NOT USED IN AN ATTEMPT TO CONTROL ONGOING EPISODES.

CORTICOSTEROIDS

These are the most powerful agents available for the treatment of a variety of respiratory disorders, including asthma. They are endogenous substances released by the adrenal cortex and have important physiological effects on many organs: A deficiency of these hormones may result in death. When used in pharmacological doses, many of the undesired effects of corticosteroids are simply an amplification of their normal physiological actions.

Corticosteroids are nonspecific in action; thus, their ability to serve as a potent anti-inflammatory agent with a number of disorders. On the other hand, the nonspecificity of their action is associated with two potential problems: (a) the normal mechanism for combating infections is suppressed, thus increasing the likelihood of acquiring serious infections; and (b) since corticosteroid therapy is palliative and symptoms are suppressed, the cause and potential progress of the underlying disease may not be specifically addressed by either the physician or the patient.

Cortisol is synthesized and secreted by the adrenal cortex under the stimulatory action of adrenocorticotropic hormone (ACTH) which is released from the anterior pituitary gland. ACTH production is stimulated when the corticosteroid level decreases to a point and activates the hypothalamus to release corticotropin-releasing factor, which stimulates the release of ACTH from the pituitary.

ACTIONS OF STEROIDS

1. Their anti-inflammatory action, and especially their ability to decrease the release of mediators in the areas of inflammation.

2. Their effectiveness in severe asthma because of their ability to abolish the tachyphylaxis that may develop to both inhaled and subcutaneous beta-adrenergic agonists, thus potentiating the effects of beta-agonists on bronchial smooth muscles.

3. Other actions include their ability to:

    a. Potentiate the response to beta-agonists both by influencing the function properties of the beta-adrenergic receptor and by increasing the number of these receptors;

    b. Inhibit arachidonic acid metabolite production;

    c. Decrease mucus production;

    d. Inhibit basophil mediator release;

    e. Reduce histamine synthesis;

    f. Suppress binding of IgE by Fc receptors; and

    g. Produce vasoconstriction.

MECHANISM OF ACTION OF GLUCOCORTICOIDS

Immunosuppressive and Anti-Inflammatory Effects

Affects cellular elements;

Inhibits delayed hypersensitivity reactions;

Produces vasoconstriction of inflamed vessels--blocks release, synthesis, and actions of permeability-increasing agents such as histamine, platelet-activating factor, prostaglandin D2, leukotriene D4, bradykin;

Affects lipid mediators--decreases synthesis of prostaglandins and leukotrienes; and

Inhibits chemotaxis at suprapharmacological concentrations.

Effect on Beta-Adrenergic Receptor Responsiveness

Abolishes the tachyphylaxis to beta-adrenergic agents.

Effects on Cellular Metabolism

Stimulates hepatic gluconeogenesis;

Decreases peripheral utilization of glucose;

Increases protein catabolism;

Increases lipolysis; and

Exerts a "permissive effect" for the metabolic action of other hormones.

Miscellaneous Effects

Inhibits fibroblast growth and collagen synthesis;

Decreases reticuloendothelial clearance of antibody-coated cells;

Mildly decreases immunoglobulin levels, but does not decrease specific antibody production; and

Decreases lysosomal release and stabilization of lysosomal membranes at suprapharmacological concentrations.

INDICATIONS FOR STEROID USE

1. With severe asthma, including: (a) acute asthma; (b) status asthmaticus; and (c) chronic asthma.

2. Self-limiting asthmatic flare-ups.

3. Prevention of adrenal insufficiency.

4. Diagnostic purposes.

METHODS OF ADMINISTRATION

Going from most to least preferable, the modes of taking corticosteroids would be: (a) inhaled; (b) every other morning; (c) every day; and (d) twice or more a day.

1. There are three forms of inhaled steroids:

    a. Beclomethasone Dipropionate (BDP): This medication, brand names Vanceril® and Beclovent®, was approved for use in 1976. The effectiveness of BDP is dose related. The usual adult dose is 400 mcg/day, but 1,000 mcg/day may be required in some patients. Mild adrenal suppression may be seen at doses greater than 1600 mcg/day. BDP is recommended to be given in divided doses 3 to 4 times each day, although in some patients with mild asthma, twice a day doses may be as effective.

    b. Triamcinolone acetonide (TAA)(A nonpolar, water-insoluble fluorinated steroid): A TAA metered-dose inhaler, brand name AeroBid®, is packaged with a special spacer delivery system designed to minimize disposition of the drug in the oral cavity. One puff releases approximately 200 ug of TAA, of which approximately 100 ug of the drug is delivered to the airways. The recommended daily dose is 2 puffs 3 to 4 times a day; TAA has been shown to be effective for mild-to-moderate asthma in both short-term and long-term studies.

    c. Flunisolide: This medication, brand name Azmacort®, is approximately equal to TAA in anti-inflammatory potency. Approximately 30 to 40% of the inhaled dose of flunisolide is absorbed and then rapidly degraded to inactive metabolites. The recommended starting dose is 2 puffs twice a day with each puff delivering about 250 ug to the airway.

2. Alternate-day oral therapy: Side-effects are reduced with this procedure; thus, it is recommended over daily steroids. Alternate-day therapy is associated with less or no suppression of fever, white blood cell counts, or delayed-type hypersensitivity skin tests.

3. Daily oral therapy: It should be given in a single dose in the morning. In most cases, this is equivalent to several divided doses during the day. Since side-effects are related primarily to the total dosage and duration of therapy, oral daily corticosteroids should be administered for the shortest period and at the lowest therapeutic dose possible.

TABLE 2:5. ADVERSE SIDE EFFECTS OF CORTICOSTEROIDS

Probable side effects:
1. Cushingoid habitus;
2. Osteoporosis;
3. Subcapsular cataracts;
4. Growth retardation in children;
5. Increased appetite; and
6. Dermal atrophy, increased fragility and striae.

Possible side effects:
1. Peptic ulcer disease;
2. Hypertension;
3. Glucose intolerance;
4. Increased risk of opportunistic infection;
5. CNS manifestations--mood alterations (euphoria, depression), pseudotumor cerebri, psychosis;
6. Avascular necrosis; and
7. Steroid myopathy.

Side effects that occur with inhaled steroids:

1. Thrush; and
2. Dysphoria.

Side effects that occur with oral steroids:
1. Weight gain, mood change, ulcers, gastrointestinal bleeding, osteoporosis, diabetes, hypertension, growth, and adrenal suppression.

ANTICHOLINERGIC DRUGS

The use of anticholinergic drugs grew out of herbal medicine. Three centuries ago, the medical literature of India recommended smoking the leaves of plants that contain anticholinergic drugs. Other plants, including deadly nightshade, jimson weed, locoweed, stink weed, thorn apple, devil's apple, and henbane, were widely smoked, chewed, and drunk to treat asthma throughout Europe and North America in the 19th century. These herbs continue to be used today because of their low cost and ready availability.

Recent years have reestablished the efficacy of anticholinergic drugs in reversing bronchoconstriction. Newer compounds--ipratropium bromide and atropine methonitrate--dilate airways effectively and have almost no significant adverse effects in therapeutic doses.

TABLE 2:6.   ANTICHOLINERGIC AND BETA-ADRENERGIC DRUGS

Situations where anticholinergic drugs may be preferred to beta-adrenergic drugs:

1. If beta-adrenergic agonists cause severe tremor;
2. If a patient tolerates tachycardia poorly (ipratropium may be used);
3. In treating attacks precipitated by beta-adrenergic blockers; and
4. In treating attacks precipitated by cholinesterase inhibitors.

Possible benefits of combined therapy with anticholinergic and beta-adrenergic drugs:

1. Increase the duration of action of one nebulized treatment;
2. Cause fewer adverse effects if each drug is used in lower concentrations than it is in single drug therapy; and
3. Have greater bronchodilator effect than either drug used alone in maximal dosage.

LESS COMMONLY USED ASTHMA MEDICATIONS

ANTIHISTAMINES

1. Antihistamines may be prescribed to dry up a post nasal drip that could trigger an asthma episode.

2. Newer antihistamines appear to have a bronchodilating effect in people with asthma. These medications also do not produce the sleepiness associated with older antihistamine compounds.

3. A potential problem with antihistamines is that they have been implicated in the drying up of mucus; this event, in turn, could result in airway closing. When a worsening of their asthma occurs when taking antihistamines, patients should notify their physicians.

DECONGESTANTS

1. Three oral decongestants, present in over-the-counter or prescriptive medications, may control nasal and sinus symptoms associated with asthma. The decongestants are: (a) pseudoephedrine, found in Sudafed® and Novafed®; (b) phenylpropanolamine, often found in combination preparations or Entex®; and (c) phenylephrine.

2. Potential problems with these drugs are that they may accentuate the side effects, such as nervousness, nausea, and headache, that may accompany the taking of asthma medications.

ANTI-MUCUS AGENTS

Expectorants or agents that react with mucus have limited value in treating patients with asthma. Potassium iodine, however, may be a useful expectorant if used for only short periods of time.

ANTIBIOTICS

1. These are useful with patients who have bacterial infections that complicate an original viral infection, or for patients who produce considerable mucus.

2. Antibiotics may also be useful in treating a sinus infection, such as sinusitis, if secretions are dripping from the nose into the lung and precipitating asthma attacks.

3. Finally, antibiotics have a place in the treatment of agents grown from sputum, such as forms of pneumonia or influenza.

TROLEANDOMYCIN (TAO)

1. This antibiotic interacts with methylprednisolone (Medrol®) in such a way that there could be a steroid-sparing effect. The latter might reduce the amount of steroids taken by patients with asthma.

2. The medication makes the lungs less hyperreactive, another reason it might be prescribed in the treatment of asthma.

3. On the negative side, it is important to perform periodic liver function tests on patients given TAO. In addition, if too much TAO is given or if the dose of Medrol® is not tapered rapidly enough, there could be an increase in steroid side effects.

CALCIUM CHANNEL BLOCKERS

1. Two calcium blocking agents have been studied for their role as an asthma drug: nifedipine (Procardia Adalet®) and verapamil (Calen Isoptin®). The agents do not open the airways, but they can be used in the treatment of medical conditions where the alternative agent counteracts adrenalin and produces airway obstruction.

METHOTREXATE

1. This drug has potential in producing significant improvement in asthmatic symptoms despite the lowering of the steroid dose. It also has minimal side effects.

GOLD

1. Gold therapy, often used in the treatment of arthritis, has proven useful with certain asthmatic patients in that it may permit a decrease in steroid requirements.

CONTROVERSIAL (AND GENERALLY WORTHLESS) APPROACHES TO THE TREATMENT OF ASTHMA

Because asthma is such a mystery both to patients and to those who treat it, a number of controversial approaches have been suggested for treatment of the disorder. The only rationale for any success of these approaches, recently summarized in an excellent chapter by Selner (1990), is because of what is referred to as superstitious behavior. This principle states that events that have absolutely no relationship are somehow connected in a person's thinking. Think of the old line, "Step on a crack, break your mother's back." How many of us actually avoided stepping on cracks in order to save the health of our mothers? (We won't ask for a show of hands--it could be embarrassing!) Anyhow, you know the process; unfortunately, it has caused asthmatic patients endless grief because worthless treatments have often been linked to an amelioration with a patient's asthma. Those noted by Selner (1990) include:

1. Subcutaneous or sublingual provocation testing.

This procedure entails injecting or placing under the tongue minute quantities of foods or chemicals that will supposedly provoke virtually any symptom. There is no evidence that the procedure achieves this aim although, as Selner (1990) notes, large quantities of a substance to which a patient is allergic might induce a generalized reaction such as an analphylactic seizure.

2. Orthomolecular medicine.

There is no evidence that the indiscriminate use of vitamins, trace elements, or glandular substances have a role in the treatment of asthma. This should not preclude, cautioned Selner (1990), continuing inquiries into the use of Vitamin C and Vitamin B6 in legitimate medical trials that could show a role for these vitamins in the treatment of asthma.

3. Acupuncture.

Despite claims to the contrary, applying needles to points of the body has not been shown to benefit the patient with asthma.

4. Herbal medicine.

There is no evidence that herbs are useful in treating asthma. On the other hand, some herbal medications can be toxic, including sassafras, chamomile, ginseng, and alfalfa seeds.

5. Chiropractic practices.

Manipulations of the body, outside of postural drainage, have not been shown to alter asthma. The same can be said about other chiropractic practices, including: (a) colonic purges to eliminate toxins from the body; (b) modification of the so-called Ehrlander technique where a patient holds a glass container in one hand and a chiropractor identifies specific organ abnormalities; (c) auto urine injection whereby urine obtained from the asthmatic patient is injected under his or her skin or intramuscularly; (d) electracupuncture, sometimes referred to as electrodiagnosis, electrodermal response testing, autogenic response testing, or Voll testing; and (e) iridology, whereby elaborate schemes have been developed which claim to identify certain areas of the body and relate them to locations on the iris of the eye.

6. Chelation therapy.

This involves the binding of a metal ion by a molecule of a specific chemical. The approach involves patients spending time in a sauna to sweat chemicals out of their bodies; at the same time, a number of supplements are given the patient which are claimed to mobilize the chemicals out of the tissues. There is no specific validity to this approach.

7. Mega amounts of Vitamin C.

The problem here is not only that Vitamin C has not been proven to have a role in the treatment of asthma, but that the patient can actually take a toxic dose of Vitamin C believing that it will help his or her asthma.

8. Hair analysis.

There is no value to the reputed analysis by a computer of hair supplied by a patient with asthma.

9. Yeast.

According to this theory, yeast overgrowth is responsible for asthma. There is no evidence, however, to support this claim.

10. Carrying around a Chihuahua dog.

This is one of our favorites: Because they make a wheezing-like sound when they breathe, it has long been thought, particularly in the Southwest, that carrying around a Chihuahua dog could benefit the patient with asthma. The rationale was that because the dog's breathing and asthma sound alike, there would somehow be a magical transference of symptoms from the patient to the dog. There is no scientific basis for this action; if anything, dander from the dog could exacerbate the asthma of patients allergic to dog dander.

References

Atkins, F. M. (1987). Use of cromolyn in asthma. Seminars in Respiratory Medicine, 8, 381-386.

Bethel, R. A., & Irvin, C. G. (1987). Anticholinergic drugs and asthma. Seminars in Respiratory Medicine, 8, 366-371.

Clark, T. J. H. (1985). Inhaled corticosteroid therapy: A substitute for theophylline as well as prednisolone? Journal of Allergy & Clinical Immunology, 75, 330-334.

Fernandez, E. (1987) Beta-adrenergic agonists. Seminars in Respiratory Medicine, 8, 353-365.

Hill, M. R. & Szefler, S. J. (1987). Theophylline update: Current controversies. Seminars in Respiratory Medicine, 8, 372-380.

Hollister, J. R. & Bowyer, S. L. (1987). Adverse side-effects of corticosteroids. Seminars in Respiratory Medicine, 8, 400-405.

Kaliner, M., Eggleston, P. A., & Mathews, K. P. (1987). Rhinitis and asthma. JAMA, 258, 2851-2873.

King, T. E., & Chang, S. W. (1987). Corticosteroid therapy in the management of asthma. Seminars in Respiratory Medicine, 8, 387-399.

Plaut, T. F. (1988). Children with Asthma: A Manual for Parents. Amherst, MA: Pedipress, Inc.

Selner, J. (1990). Controversial approaches to the treatment of asthma and allergic disease: What to watch out for. In S. Spector & N. Sander (Eds.) Understanding Asthma: A Blueprint for Breathing, 175-183. Palatine, IL: American College of Allergy & Immunology.

Spector, S. (1990). Day-to-day management of asthma. In S. Spector & N. Sander (Eds.) Understanding Asthma: A Blueprint for Breathing, 37-62. Palatine, IL: American College of Allergy & Immunology.

<u>XANTHINE MEDICATIONS</u>
VISUAL 2.1

Generic Types
Theophylline, aminophylline, dyphylline,
and oxtriphylline

Mode of Action
Relaxes smooth muscles in the airways

Dosage Forms
Orally, intravenously, rectally

Therapeutic Blood Levels

Side Effects
Transient: nausea, nervousness
More serious: stomach acidity, gastrointestinal problems, confusion, convulsions, hives, stomach cramps, rapid breathing/heartbeat, vomiting blood

Interactions
Decreased blood levels: tobacco/marijuana
smoking, charcoal broiled foods, anticonvulsant
drugs, high protein/low carbohydrate diet
Increased blood levels: cimetidine, fever, low
protein/high carbohydrate diet, propranolol,
allopurinol, certain antibiotics (e.g.,
erythromycin)

ADRENERGIC BRONCHODILATORS
VISUAL 2.2

Generic Types

Albuterol, ephedrine, epinephrine, terbutaline, metaproterenol, isoetharine, ethynorepinephrine, isoproterenol, bifolterol mesylate

Mode of Action

Relaxes smooth muscles of the airways

Dosage Forms

Oral, inhaled, injection

Side Effects

Transient: dizziness, headache, increased blood pressure, nausea/vomiting, nervousness, disturbed sleep, increased sweating, weakness

More serious: chest pain, irregular heartbeat

CROMOLYN SODIUM
VISUAL 2.3

Mode of Action

Inhibits the production and release of
substances that mediate allergic
reactions in the lungs
Lessens lung response to allergic triggers
Can prevent but not treat narrowed airways

Dosage Forms

Inhaled

Effectiveness

1-3 month trial

Side Effects

Minor/transient: cough, harseness
More serious: chest pain, chills, difficult
urination, dizziness, persistent
headache, increased wheezing/chest
tightness, swollen joints, muscle pain,
nausea/vomiting, skin rashes, unusual
sweating

CORTICOSTEROIDS
VISUAL 2.4

Generic Types
Prednisone, prednisolone,
methylprednisolone, triamcinolone,
B-methasone, dexamethasone,
hydrocortisone, cortisone,
beclamethasone, flunisolide,
triamcinolone, acetonide

Mode of Action
Decreases inflammation and reduces
swelling and allergic reactions in the
lungs
Some relaxation of bronchial smooth
muscle, dilated airways

Dosage Forms
Oral, inhaled, intravenous, injection

Side Effects
Minor: Oral yeast infections with inhaled
steroids
Major: Changes in body shape
Adrenal suppression
Reduced growth rate

ANTICHOLINERGIC BRONCHODILATORS
VISUAL 2.5

Generic Types
Ipratropium bromide

Mode of Action
Inhibits acetylcholine, a messenger in the nervous system, thereby blocking vagus nerve mediated bronchoconstriction

Dosage Form
Inhaled

Side Effects
Rare: Cough

Very rare: Nervousness, nausea, gastrointestinal distress, and dry mouth

SELF-MANAGEMENT AND MEDICATIONS
VISUAL 2.6

1. Take medications exactly as prescribed.

2. Take maintenance medications even when feeling well.

3. Report suspected side effects to your physician.

4. Be aware of drug interactions that may decrease the effectiveness of your medications.

5. Clean your metered-dose inhalers to ensure proper functioning and to prevent oral infections.

6. Learning the proper mechanics for using inhalers will make certain you are receiving an effective dose of medication.

7. Overuse of inhaled adrenergic bronchodilators during an attack can worsen the episode.

8. Cromolyn should not be used during an attack.

9. Cromolyn must be taken regularly for 1 to 3 months before effects are usually seen.

10. When using inhaled steroids, gargle with water to prevent fungal infections.

11. Do not use inhaled steroids during an attack; they may worsen the episode.

12. Do not stop oral steroids (pill form) suddenly.

13. Overuse or dependence on inhalers may result in underuse of other asthma management strategies, leading to serious asthma episodes.

IMMUNOTHERAPY
VISUAL 2.7

Mode of Action
50% of adult asthmatics have allergy-induced asthma
Alters immunologic reactivity of allergic individual

When Is Immunotherapy Indicated?
Medications fail to control allergy induced asthma
Skin tests
Blood tests
Inhalation challenge tests

Dosage
Shots of increasing dosage
1-2 shots per week, frequency decreased over 4-6 months to
monthly maintenance dose

Side Effects
Mild: Itching, hives, local reactions
Serious: Systemic reaction, anaphylactic shock

Effectiveness
Most useful for treatment of allergies to dust, mites, grass
and animal dander
Effectiveness seen within 6 months usually
Old or new allergies may (re)appear after shots discontinued

SESSION THREE
ASTHMA PREVENTION

GOALS

1. Discuss factors and problems associated with medication noncompliance.

2. Teach patients to identify or recognize their asthma triggers and outline ways to avoid and/or cope with them.

3. Teach patients how to identify the early warning signs of their asthma.

EQUIPMENT

Name tags.
Paper and pencils for all participants.
Overhead projector or slide projector.
Blackboard or grease pen and blank sheets for overhead.

SUPPLIES

Coffee, tea, snacks, or light lunch.

SESSION THREE OUTLINE

TOPIC/ ACTIVITY	REQUIRED MATERIAL	APPROXIMATE TIME ALLOWED
Welcome & salutations	Name tags	5 minutes
Questions about prior sessions/readings		10 minutes
Medication compliance discussion	Visual 3.1	15 minutes
Asthma triggers discussion	Visual 3.2	25 minutes
Asthma early warning signs discussion	Visual 3.3, Early Warning Signs Worksheet (Handout 2.1)	25 minutes
Open discussion		10 minutes
Homework	SOLVED Problems Exercise focused on medication compliance or asthma triggers, Visual 3.4, read Chapter 5	10 minutes

SESSION THREE TEACHING NOTES

Welcome and Salutations

Provide a name tag for each participant. Allow time for small talk among group members prior to introducing the session material.

Questions About Prior Sessions/Readings

Allow the group time to ask questions about material covered earlier in the program.

Medication Compliance

Have the group brainstorm about reasons for not taking medications as prescribed (i.e., in the right dose and on the right schedule). Noncompliance factors can be listed on the board. Use Visual 3.1 to help fill in noncompliance factors not addressed by the group.

Asthma Triggers

Have the group generate as many asthma triggers as possible, with the leader grouping triggers into classes on the board (e.g., allergens, irritants, mechanical factors). Complete the trigger list using Visual 3.2. Next, have the group brainstorm coping strategies or self-management behaviors appropriate for dealing with each class of trigger. The group leader might use Visual 3.2, and cover up the recommended coping strategies until the group has responded.

Early Warning Signs of Asthma

Rely on the group to report their own early warning signs prior to presenting the complete list on the Early Warning Signs outline. Help the group distinguish between physical, behavioral, and emotional signs.

Open Discussion

Allow a period of open discussion on asthma prevention before the session has ended.

Homework

Reintroduce the SOLVED Problems Exercise and instruct the participants to apply this exercise to a problem of their choice. Encourage the participants to focus on medication compliance, asthma triggers, or problems they encounter in recognizing early warning signs. Ask the participants to read Chapter Five before next session.

SESSION THREE BACKGROUND READING

ASTHMA PREVENTION

SELF-STATEMENTS AND THE PREVENTION OF ASTHMA ATTACKS

Specific methods have been presented which may assist a patient to prevent or avoid asthma. This section will augment this discussion by describing the role of self-statements in this process. Our use of language provides us with the ability to generate statements to direct our actions. The statements patients make to themselves, for example, can allow them not only to help prevent and avoid attacks, but to manage both asthmatic episodes and the consequences of asthma.

Self-statements are the remarks we make to ourselves to prompt, direct, change, or maintain behavior (O'Leary & Dubey, 1979). There are two types: self-instructions and beliefs. They are considered among the most powerful influences in affecting our behavior (Watson & Tharp, 1989). We use self-statements from the moment we awake and tell ourselves to get out of bed until we tell ourselves it is time to turn out the light and go to sleep. In between, we constantly use self-instruction, from guiding ourselves through the traffic of a busy city to working through possible alternatives we have to solve day-to-day problems. Self-statements are useful not only in acquiring skills for the self-management of asthma, but in the later performance of these skills in attempting to control the disorder. Self-statements can be especially effective if they permit the patient to prevent an unnecessary attack. The latter consequence, when resulting from the patient's behavior, can be self-reinforcing; he or she will likely use similar self-instruction in the future in attempts to avoid asthma flare-ups.

There are three factors which increase the effectiveness of self-statements:

1. **They are particularly effective when used frequently by patients.** If patients are repeatedly able to prompt and direct their behavior so as to avoid attacks, it will increase the probability they will use such statements in the future. This reinforcement of behavior, especially when it occurs in the natural environment, is essential for the self-management of asthma.

2. **The level of performance of self-management skills increases with performance induced by self-instruction.** Patients not only refine their skills, but they acquire positive expectations concerning the probable outcomes of their actions.

3. **Self-statements are often more effective than externally-imposed instructions in managing behavior.** We would rather do what we tell ourselves than what others tell us to do. When patients prompt themselves to act in accordance with medical instructions for managing their asthma, they make a significant contribution to the overall control of the disorder.

There are a number of types of self-statements patients use which can help control asthma. Included here would be: (a) establishing self-determined goals; (b) self-assessment; (c) self-reinforcement; (d) making any changes in plans for achieving goals; and (e) self-directed stimulus control. Each of these functions will be discussed separately.

A.   Establishing self-determined goals.

      Self-determined goals help focus our attention and provide instruction. When combined
with reinforcement we provide ourselves for successfully performing a task and achieving a
goal, they are as effective as externally controlled criteria; they prompt us to seek reaching
the goal more frequently in the future.

      Watson and Tharp (1989) have suggested eight tactics for establishing self-goals
(Table 3:1). All are relevant to the management of asthma.

TABLE 3:1.   EIGHT TACTICS TO USE IN SETTING SELF-GOALS

(Suggested by Watson & Tharp, 1989)

Make a list of concrete examples.

List the aspects of behavior that you want to control.

Become an observer of yourself.

Strive to increase desirable behaviors.

Specify chain of events that produce a goal.

Observe those who do what you want to do. Model their behavior.

Think of alternative solutions.

Realize that reaching a goal requires chaining certain of your
      behaviors.

---

1. Make a list of concrete examples.

      Rather than start with some vague statement such as, "I want to control my asthma,"
it is better to compile a series of specific behaviors that the patient can perform. These
might include, "I will comply with medication instructions;" "I will pay attention and
try to avoid stimuli I know cause my attacks;" and "I will pay attention to early warning
signals of my asthma and begin treating an attack when it is still mild." Attaining these
goals will help the patient control his or her asthma.

2.   The patient should list the aspects of his or her asthma that he or she is attempting to
      control.

      In order to manage the disorder, the patient must attend to details. Questions the
patient may wish to ask include: "Where do the majority of my attacks occur?" " What
factors seem to precede these episodes?" and "What are the consequences of my asthma?"

The patient should make a list of these details and then select what seem the most crucial factors to control. Often, an idea of events surrounding an attack are unclear; jotting down specifics will clarify many particulars about asthma for the patient. These details can not only provide the patient with more information about managing his or her attacks, but they also can help change the patient's beliefs and expectations about his or her ability to achieve this goal.

3. Become an observer of oneself.

There is not much need to dwell upon this topic--self-monitoring is a topic stressed throughout Asthma Self-Management. Watson and Tharp (1989) emphasize an aspect of self-management which should be repeated: In order to learn about events surrounding an attack, the patient must stop speculating about events, and start observing the behavior and the context within which attacks occur. There are various degrees of observation; practice at observation increases the patient's knowledge about the behavior and decreases the tendency to speculate about events.

4. The patient should always strive to increase desirable behaviors.

Even if the patient wishes to decrease a behavior, such as worrying about his or her asthma, the best approach is to solve the problem by focusing on a desirable alternative behavior. For example, instead of worrying, the patient can specify the steps he or she knows and can perform to help manage attacks. By repeatedly practicing such skills, the patient increases a desirable behavior; this performance, in turn, should reduce the undesirable response of worrying about asthma.

5. Specify the chain of events that will produce a goal.

The events that comprise an asthma attack can often be conceived of as a chain. A typical chain would include the setting where the attack occurs, the stimulus that triggers the flare-up, the physical reaction that constitutes the attack, and, most significant from the point of view of self-management, the chain of responses made by the patient to bring the episode under control. Instruction in learning and performing chains of behaviors to manage attacks is at the core of Asthma Self-Management.

6. The patient should observe people who efficaciously do what he or she wants to do and then try it.

When the patient suffers asthma, particularly if hospitalized, he or she has the opportunity to see how others manage flare-ups. The patient should pay particular attention to the performance of patients who manage their asthma well; there is a considerable amount of knowledge that can be transmitted by imitating others. It is always wise to observe how patients manage their asthma and not rely entirely upon what they say they do (even though such accounts are often accurate). In addition, examples in Asthma Self-Management suggest numerous ways to manage attacks. The patient should constantly review and practice these methods; they can later be of immense help in bringing an asthmatic episode under control.

7. Think of alternative solutions.

As the patient becomes skilled at observing his or her behavior, the patient may realize that the strategies adopted are not effective in the management of his or her asthma. The patient may wish to review all of the techniques that have been taught in Asthma Self-Management; jotting them down on a list can help in this review. The patient may wish to use the process of brainstorming to develop the best possible strategy for the future management of attacks. Brainstorming involves four simple rules: (a) initially trying for quantity in thinking of all potential solutions they have been taught--quality of ideas will follow this process; (b) do not be critical of the ideas generated--criticism of specific ideas will follow; (c) be freewheeling in considering the procedures taught; and (d) try to improve procedures by combining them (Watson & Tharp, 1989).

8. Even if the goal is not a specific behavior, reaching the goal will require changing certain behaviors.

The goal of a self-management program for asthma is to establish as much control as possible by the patient over the disorder. This requires that the patient learn and perform the behaviors taught throughout Asthma Self-Management. There will be changes and an evolution of goals as the patient progresses through the program. Initially, the patient may lack both the knowledge of the skills and the confidence to perform these skills to manage attacks. With practice, however, the patient's goals will change so that he or she may come not only to be skilled at performing self-management skills, but wish to be as effective as possible in using these techniques in preventing or managing an asthma attack.

B. Self-assessment.

This is the key to the successful application of self-management procedures for asthma. If used alone, it often does not produce change (O'Leary & Dubey, 1979); if combined with other procedures, such as the performance of self-management skills, it becomes significant. It is also an important ingredient in self-reinforcement because it permits the patient to know when to reward him/herself for successfully executing skills that prevent or manage asthma attacks.

Much of the self-observation conducted in Asthma Self-Management centers around the diaries, report of attack forms, and other structured paper-and-pencil instruments. These instruments serve as handy guides for the patient to assist in selecting the behaviors to be observed and information recorded about. Patients should consider the ABCs of observation. These include:

1. Antecedents (A).

The major questions that the patient wants to consider, in analyzing any asthmatic flare-up, are:

a. When did the attack occur?

b. Who was the patient with when the episode occurred?

c. What was the patient doing?

d. Where was the patient?

e. How did the patient respond to the attack?

Answers to all these questions provide a considerable amount of information, as well as avoiding needless speculation, about events that surround in an asthma attack. This knowledge will be sought by an experienced physician; the information, however, can be equally important to the patient in successfully utilizing self-management skills to control asthma.

2. Behaviors (B).

Included here would be the patient's actions, thoughts, and feelings. It would be important not only to know the type of actions taken to manage the episode, but the patient's thoughts and feelings about the flare-up, e.g., "I was scared, but confident that I could manage the episode." Since the patient is the only individual actually experiencing these thoughts and feelings, he or she must accurately report such data on the paper-and-pencil instruments used throughout Asthma Self-Management.

3. Consequences (C).

This would include data on such factors as what happened as a result of the patient's actions, as well as feelings about the outcome. Such information is often experienced only by the patient; for this reason, it is imperative to note the consequences of his or her actions on one of the structured data forms used in Asthma Self-Management.

There are a number of problems that can arise in self-assessment. Those which should be avoided include:

a. Waiting too long to record observations. The longer the delay between observations and the recording of this information, the greater the likelihood that either erroneous information will be recorded or important data will be omitted. Thus, the need to complete diary forms daily and the completion of a report form immediately following an attack or episode.

b. Collecting inaccurate information. There are times when the patient may be so concerned about pleasing others that he or she knowingly or unknowingly enters inaccurate data on structured forms in Asthma Self-Management. It must be repeatedly emphasized that accurate information be recorded; inaccurate data only cheat the patient by his or her failing to make adjustments in the program or to provide additional training to the patient.

c. Patient discouragement. If the patient fails to perceive changes between actions and the severity of the asthma, the patient may become discouraged and feel that self-management skills are inappropriate for the condition. Constant support of patients is a hallmark of successful self-management programs (Kanfer, 1980). Constant support allows time to make adjustments in the self-management skills taught, while keeping the patient motivated to record accurate information about his or her asthma.

d. Do not record information in an automatic way. After awhile, all patients more or less adept at observing and recording information about themselves. Unfortunately, some patients may make the process too automatic and absentmindedly record information. The problem that arises is that the data may be inaccurate. A way to keep this common problem from occurring is to: (1) obtain data only during prescribed periods of time and not continuously throughout the program; and (2) periodically review the importance of record keeping.

e. Observe and record information about certain aspects of behavior. An advantage of structured recording instruments is that patients attend only to aspects of their behavior as requested on the forms. When this process does not occur, patients may try to attend to too much of their responding; the result, in this case, is usually unreliable information.

f. Reactivity. This is usually a positive outcome in that the patient may begin to change behavior in a positive direction in accordance with the categories of information requested on the structured forms. For example, many patients begin to comply to medication instructions when requested to monitor such behavior. However, the danger is that the patient may try and change too many behaviors at once; this approach, in turn, can result in patient failure and subsequent disenchantment with the program. Thus, the caveat to patients is to try and change one behavior at a time; this approach, basically involving shaping, can result in achieving the final goal--the self-management of asthma without encountering personal failure.

g. Overreactivity by patients to their behaviors. There are times when, if asked to record information about certain responses, the patient becomes preoccupied with the effort and pays too much attention to the responses. There is no better example than attending too much to breathing. Breathing is an automatic response; however, it is a response that, when attended to, can be inadvertently altered. The patient may think that he or she is experiencing asthma when a breathing change is due to other ˉ factors such as exercise; or, he or she may fail to perceive an incipient attack, believing his or her breathing is normal (Creer, 1983). Either possibility should be avoided.

C. Self-reinforcement.

Self-reinforcement entails that each patient select a reinforcer that is personally desirable so he or she might establish it as a contingency for the performance of self-management skills. Depending upon the goals established by the patient in performing these skills, the patient can then decide if the performance attains these goals and should be reinforced.

There are three general principles to the use of self-reinforcement in self-management (e.g., Watson & Tharp, 1989). These are:

1. Discovering and selecting a reinforcer.

Through contemplation and direct observation, a patient can write down what seems important to him. What reinforcers would he or she work for and use as a contingency as a reward for performing self-management techniques? What object does he or she want and is willing to delay receiving contingent upon performance? Every patient will have a different list. Many will prove impractical because, while many people might like a Porsche, it is not economically feasible. Wherever possible, the patient should be encouraged to use activities as reinforcers. These are especially effective when placed in the context of Premack's Principle. Basically, this principle is based upon the assumption that any activity you are likely to perform can serve as a reinforcer for any behavior that you are less likely to perform. This sounds complicated, but it is not. Most of us would like to spend time watching our favorite program on television or reading a good novel. However, we may know that we also must perform some activity, such as cleaning up the bathroom or completing homework. To use Premack's Principle effectively, we tell ourselves that we will watch our favorite TV program only if we first clean up the bathroom. In this respect, viewing the TV program has now become contingent upon our first attaining a sparkling clean bathroom. This simple principle is very important to self-reinforcement: it provides us with an effective technique to manage our own behavior.

2. Knowledge and reinforcement.

Once the patient has established the contingencies between a selected reinforcer and behavior, he or she then has to teach him/herself to become aware of the performance of that behavior so that it can be reinforced. In short, the patient behaves, then reinforces him/herself. Knowing when to reinforce oneself for appropriate contingent behavior provides information to the patient. The patient learns when and under what circumstances to behave in an appropriate manner. This information, in turn, should strengthen the performance of self-management skills in the control of asthma.

3. Delivery of self-reinforcement.

Self-reinforcement appears to obey other laws of reinforcement. The important laws to consider include:

a. Reinforce immediately or as soon as possible. As soon as the patient performs a response that is contingent upon reinforcement, he or she should reinforce himself or herself. This will strengthen the behavior or response.

b. Start out by reinforcing oneself each time the contingent behavior is performed. After the behavior is well-established, the patient will wish to switch to an intermittent schedule. This may involve reinforcement after a prescribed period of time or after a certain number of behaviors have been performed; the schedule may also be variable or fixed. The reason for switching from reinforcing every response to reinforcing after a certain number of responses or a certain period of time is that behaviors are strongest when rewarded under these reinforcement schedules. In other words, the patient is more apt to continue performing self-management skills after he or she has reinforced himself or herself for such performance on an intermittent schedule.

c. There are times when the patient is unable to reinforce himself or herself until a
    later time. When this occurs, the patient may wish to use one of two techniques (or
    both) as a bridge between performance and reinforcement. The two techniques are:
    (1) self-statements, where the patient verbally reinforces himself or herself for
    successfully performing self-management skills, and (2) imagery, where the
    patient imagines that he or she is reinforcing himself or herself for successful
    performance of these skills.

D. Making necessary plans and changes.

The self-management skills stressed in Asthma Self-Management are designed to assist
patients to cope with and help control their asthma. Within the guidelines of this program,
the patient may have other goals that he or she wishes to attain. For example, as part of a
health care regimen, the patient may wish to exercise more each day. There are a number of
general suggestions that have been offered for planning and implementing self-management
programs for specific target behaviors (Table 3:2). The general strategies we will review
are suggested by Martin and Pear (1988) and Watson and Tharp (1989).

TABLE 3:2. GENERAL STRATEGIES FOR PLANNING THE IMPLEMENTING OF SELF-MANAGEMENT PROGRAMS

Specify the problem

Make a commitment to change

Make careful observations

Design a change program
  Incorporate ABC's of change

Be persistent

Be organized

Maximize social support

Maintain self-management efforts

---

1. **Specify the problem.** As noted earlier, it is always important that the patient
    specify the problem he or she is trying to correct. We will use the patient's attempt to
    increase exercise as the target behavior he or she wishes to change. Here, the patient
    does not want to set a vague and general goal, "I am going to exercise more," but wants to
    set a goal such as, "I will exercise vigorously for 20 minutes at least three times a
    week." The latter goal is specific; it will guide the patient in improving his or her
    exercise habits.

2. **Make a commitment to change.** If the patient has made a commitment to acquire the self-management skills taught through Asthma Self-Management, he or she can make a commitment to change other aspects of behavior. Without such a commitment, it would be difficult to make any behavior changes; commitment represents the motivational force that powers successful change.

3. **Make careful observations.** We stressed the importance of self-observation in an earlier section. However, it should be repeated that careful observations provide data that permit the patient to analyze the ABC relationships in behavior. As Watson and Tharp (1980) put it, careful observations permit the patient to "figure out the conditions that facilitate or compete with the target behavior" (p. 24).

4. **Design a change program.** In designing a change program, the patient not only has to consider the ABC relationships described earlier, but whether he or she needs to manage a situation, behavior, or consequences. The patient may wish to use a variety of techniques to achieve change. It may be helpful to jot down the antecedents (A), behavior (B), or consequences (C) of what he or she wishes to change. This can help formulate a change program. The patient may also wish to tinker with his or her program if performing the skills for a period has not been successful. Taking exercise as an example, the patient may move down a step and say, "I am going to exercise vigorously for 20 minutes at least twice a week." When the patient is successful at achieving this goal, he or she will then wish to increase exercising to 20 minutes three times a week. The patient may experiment with some of the techniques taught. There is no one way to change one's behavior; for this reason, the patient may tinker with any program that has been established.

5. **Be persistent.** The patient shouldn't give up just because a plan doesn't work the first time around. He or she must give it a chance to work; if it finally appears as if it is not for the patient but a faulty program, then a change should be made. In practicing the self-management skills taught to in Asthma Self-Management, knowledge and confidence will increase. Thus, there are many times when the patient may wish to improve chances of achieving goals and rearrange plans to fit his or her improved competencies more closely .

6. **Be well-organized.** In both performing self-management skills and gathering data on his or her program, the patient must be as well organized as possible. This will not only provide the patient with more accurate information about his or her efforts, but it can help in making crucial decisions as to whether or not to change the plans that are being pursued. The patient will also have the satisfaction that he or she has done well in self-monitoring and recording aspects of behavior. Reinforce the patient when this occurs!

7. **Maximize social support.** There certainly will not be a lack of support from staff members involved with Asthma Self-Management. However, it is necessary that the patient has the support of others, such as family members, if self-management skills are to be successfully performed. The patient should keep them, especially the spouse, abreast of what he or she is attempting to do to help control asthma. The patient should make family members a partner in his or her efforts; almost all of them will be more than happy to assist in this role. In addition, the patient will likely meet others in the

group who will become friends in the shared task of managing asthma. These friendships can be extremely important in that there are others who understand what the patient is going through; in addition, information can be shared, e.g., where the best buy is for asthma medications.

8. **Maintain self-management efforts.** There are often periods when the patient may wonder whether he or she need perform self-management skills; these periods are apt to be present when the patient is free of asthma. However, asthma is, as explained, an intermittent condition. Even during periods when asthma is under control and no breathing difficulty is experienced, the patient needs to follow the physician's advice and continue to monitor his or her condition. With the return of asthma flare-ups, the patient will then be ready to initiate any steps to help manage asthma.

E. Stimulus control.

This means that a response, such as an asthma attack, occurs in the presence of a particular stimulus, but not in the presence of other stimuli. Stimulus control is significant in preventing or avoiding attacks because, with some patients, the presence of a known stimulus can induce attacks. Thus, if animal dander is a trigger of attacks, the patient will want to make every effort to avoid such stimuli by staying away from dogs, cats, horses, etc. If pollution is a precipitant and pollution levels are high, the patient should listen to weather reports and remain indoors when it is noted that such counts are high and likely to produce respiratory distress. Stimulus control can also help prevent attacks in other ways; for example, the patient may wish to rearrange the way asthma medications are taken and add a stimulus which informs him or her that it is time to take a medication. A pill box with a built-in alarm is an example of a stimulus that can remind the patient to take medication.

Four guidelines are suggested by Martin and Pear (1988) to assist in establishing a discriminative stimulus to help control asthma.

1. Choosing distinctive stimuli.

If the patient is missing maintenance medications because of being too busy, he or she may wish to select a pill dispenser with a clock and an alarm to sound when medication should be taken. If the dispenser is placed in an inconspicuous place where the signal can be heard, it will help the patient to take medications as prescribed. The signals that prompt avoidance of an attack precipitant usually take the form of self-instructions. The self-statements used by the patient warn that the environment contains stimuli that may trigger asthma, and that an unnecessary attack can be prevented by removing oneself or the stimulus from the environment. Self-monitoring is especially important in assisting the patient to make such decisions.

2. Select an appropriate reinforcer.

In the section on self-reinforcement, we reviewed ways to reinforce oneself for discharging important behaviors to help prevent or avoid asthma episodes. When patients act in accordance with a discriminative stimulus that has been established, they should be certain to reinforce themselves! This will strengthen the potency of the stimulus to assist a patient in the future; it will also help strengthen the behavior occasioned by the stimulus so the reinforcer may eventually be faded out and the behavior will remain strong.

3.   Developing discrimination.

This means that the patient wants to select a distinctive stimulus as a reminder to take medication. If what is selected has a signal which sounds too much like a telephone, the patient may have difficulties in distinguishing the sounds of the pill box from that of the telephone. If the signal is entirely different from the sound of a telephone, however, this uniqueness can assist in the establishment of a discriminative stimulus. Besides establishing control over behavior, it is also imperative that the patient make self-statements about the meaning of the stimuli and the performance that it signals to perform. These self-instructions are of benefit not only in establishing the stimulus as a discriminative stimulus, but in helping to create a bridge for continuing the performance of self-management skills when the discriminative stimulus is removed. As noted above, self-instruction is likely to be the only form of stimulus control used to avoid stimuli that can precipitate attacks.

4.   Fading out the discriminative stimulus.

After awhile, the patient may find that he or she takes medication without the prompting of the discriminative stimulus. When this behavior occurs on a regular basis, the patient will want to fade the discriminative stimulus out of the environment. This may be done gradually by setting the signal to go off on an intermittent basis--say every other day--or the patient may feel that medication-taking behavior is strong enough to remove the discriminative stimulus entirely. This choice is up to the patient. Later, if he or she is beginning to miss taking maintenance medications, the discriminative stimulus may always be reinstated. The patient should never hesitate to use self-instructions for helping to avoid or prevent unnecessary asthma attacks. These self-statements, in the long run, are the most important discriminative stimuli the patient is likely to create and use to control behavior.

ALLERGIES

An allergic reaction is a series of events initiated when an allergen is introduced into the body. Allergens are stimuli that are not harmful to anyone without allergies. To those with allergies, however, these stimuli--such as mold, pollen, or animal dander--may trigger allergic reactions.

When an allergic reaction occurs, white blood cells produce IgE antibodies. These attach themselves to the "Y"-shaped IgE molecules on mast cells. The latter cells are found in the respiratory and gastrointestinal tract, as well as on the skin. When allergens and IgE molecules connect, the mast cells are activated. Potent chemicals, or mediators, are released from the mast cells; the results are the the symptoms of allergies. The best known mediator is histamine; the release of histamine causes watery eyes, runny noses, itching, and sneezing. The allergic condition asthma is triggered when allergens contact the activated mast cells located in the bronchial or breathing tubes.

TABLE 3:3. COMMON CAUSES OF ASTHMA

Kaliner (1987) recently enumerated common causes of asthma attacks. These are:

A. ALLERGIES

   1. Allergic asthma

   2. Allergic bronchopulmonary aspergillosis

B. INFECTIONS

   1. Bronchiolitis

   2. Upper respiratory tract infections

C. INDUSTRIAL-OCCUPATIONAL OR ENVIRONMENTAL STIMULI

   1. Irritants

   2. Allergens

D. CHEMICAL OR DRUG INGESTION

   1. Nonsteroidal anti-inflammatory agents, e.g., aspirin

   2. Sulfiting agents

   3. Beta-adrenergic antagonists

E. EXERCISE

F. VASCULITIS

G. IDEOPATHIC OR INTRINSIC ASTHMA

CONDITIONS THOUGHT TO EXACERBATE ASTHMA

Kaliner and colleagues (1987) listed five conditions that can exacerbate asthma:

1. Sinusitis

2. Gastroesophageal reflux

3. Pregnancy

4. Emotional and situational responses

5. Hyperthyroidism

TABLE 3:4. ENVIRONMENTAL CONTROL AND DUST ABATEMENT

The following steps should be taken by patients to control the presence of asthma triggers in the home:

1. Permit no smoking in the house.
2. Avoid strong odors, especially perfumes, aerosols, or sprays.
3. Use an exhaust fan in the kitchen while cooking.
4. Do not permit any pets in the house (except goldfish and snakes).
5. The house temperature should remain approximately 65 to 70 degrees Fahrenheit; the relative humidity should remain within 30 to 50 percent.
6. If allergic to house dust, remain out of the house during vacuuming and for several hours after vacuuming.
7. Avoid upholstered furniture or feather pillows.
8. Washable scatter rugs are preferred on floors, but synthetic rug materials and rubberized pads can be used.
9. Be certain that no mold forms in damp spaces such as bathrooms, kitchens, or in the soil and drainage pans of house plants.
10. Keep the house clean not only to prevent mold and dust, but also cockroaches. In studies, patients with asthma developed bronchospasm when exposed to an inhaled cockroach antigen.
11. Use lids on pots and exhaust fans when cooking in order to keep odors in the kitchen to a minimum.
12. Use high-efficiency particulate air filter (HEPA) systems to remove particles from the air. Electrostatic air cleaners are relatively inefficient compared to the HEPA filters.
13. Avoid feather pillows. At the same time, be aware that foam pillows can either decompose into dust or, when exposed to moisture, become a breeding ground for mold.
14. Pillows and blankets should be made of synthetic material such as Dacron polyester. They should be washed monthly and replaced yearly.
15. A mattress should be enclosed completely in plastic covers, or a waterbed can be used. Everything in the bedroom should be dustproof and washable; use plain furniture and synthetic or cotton rugs. Synthetic lightweight curtains should be used.

POTENTIAL MECHANISMS OF NOCTURNAL ASTHMA

CIRCADIAN RHYTHM: There are few data to support this factor as contributing to nocturnal asthma.

SLEEP: There are more data suggesting asthma is a sleep-associated phenomenon. In addition, the supine posture assumed during sleep has often been suspected of contributing to nocturnal asthma.

ALLERGY: There is a possibility that a patient may inhale dust or other allergens during sleep, thus leading to nocturnal asthma. However, there is little evidence for this hypothesis. Where allergy does seem to play a role in nocturnal asthma is when there is a delayed asthmatic reaction to allergen exposure that occurred during the day.

AIRWAY SECRETIONS: The overnight accumulation of mucus secretions in the airways may lead to nocturnal asthma in some patients. This is accompanied by a decrease in mucociliary clearance and the cough reflex during sleep. These mechanisms help keep the airways clear of airway secretions, including postnasal drip, that occur at night.

GASTROESOPHAGEAL REFLUX: This is defined as the flow of gastric contents across an incompetent gastroesophageal junction into the esophagus. The fluid may not only include acidic secretions of the stomach, but also duodenal juice that may have backed up in the pylorus. The supine posture taken during sleep could contribute to this problem. In addition, there is a possibility that the gastroesophageal reflux may provoke bronchoconstriction via a vagally-mediated reflex.

CIRCULATING FACTORS: Some studies have investigated corticosteroids and catecholamines as potential circulating factors. The evidence is inconclusive, however.

COMBINATION OF FACTORS: This seems to be the major finding of studies of nocturnal asthma, namely that the nocturnal worsening of asthma is the net effect of multiple contributing factors, such as those described above, and not due to a single factor.

TABLE 3:5. THERAPY FOR NOCTURNAL ASTHMA

Optimize standard therapy
    Theophylline
    Beta-adrenergics, inhaled and oral
    Bronchial hygiene

Introduce nasal or sinus treatment

Identify reversible factors

Introduce reflux regimen

Introduce course of corticosteroids

Introduce warm, humidified air

Introduce therapeutic awakenings

FOOD ALLERGIES

According to Sampson, Buckley, and Metcalf (1987), foods most commonly implicated as causing immediate hypersensitivity reactions are:

1.	Eggs	4.	Peanuts
2.	Milk	5.	White fish
3.	Tree nuts	6.	Crustacea

TABLE 3:6. AVOIDING MOLD IN FOOD

Molds form in many places, including bread or other foods, when not immediately refrigerated after use. If the patient is allergic to mold, the following precautions need to be taken:

First, always refrigerate any food that may serve as an incubator for mold. Foods included here would be bread, leftover meats, canned juices, canned vegetables, etc. Second, beware of food that contains yeast as it is conducive to the formation of mold. Finally, avoid foods and beverages that may contain mold, including:

Wine and beer	Mushrooms
Buttermilk and sour cream	Sauerkraut
Cheeses of all kinds	Smoked meats and fishes
(including cottage cheese)	Vinegar and foods
Apple cider	containing vinegar
Baked goods that contain a	Dried Fruits
large amount of yeast	

READING FOOD LABELS (suggested by Klockenbrink, 1987).

Below are some of the more widely used chemical terms that appear on food labels:

PRESERVATIVES

These include all of the preservatives added to lengthen the shelf life of food by inhibiting the growth of microorganisms or by preventing fats from breaking down and becoming rancid.

Butylated Hydroxyanisole (BHA) and Butylated Hydroxytoleuene (BHT):

1. These preservatives are antioxidants made from petroleum that prevent rancidity by retarding the decomposition of fats and oils.

2. The antioxidants are put into potato chips, vegetable oils, and processed foods such as presweetened cereals, bouillon cubes, chewing gum, and baked goods.

3. These are among the most controversial additives in that some studies indicate they cause tumors while others suggest that they prevent them.

Calcium Propionate and Sodium Propionate:

1. These preservatives are derived from propionic acid.

2. They are the additives most frequently used to prevent the growth of mold and bacteria in baked goods.

3. These preservatives are considered among the safest of food additives.

Ethylene Diamine Tetraacetic Acid (EDTA):

1. This preservative is a chelating agent that traps and removes metal contaminants introduced into foods during their manufacture.

2. EDTA can affect the taste, odor, and appearance of certain foods, such as mayonnaise, margarine, and some salad dressings and sandwich spreads.

3. EDTA can inhibit the absorption of calcium, iron, and other nutrients in the body, but is considered safe in levels permitted by the FDA.

Propyl Gallate:

1. This preservative is salt of gallic acid, which occurs naturally in tea leaves.

2. Propyl gallate is used to prevent rancidity in foods such as vegetable oils, soup mixes, potato sticks, and sandwich spreads.

3. Some concern has been voiced by consumer groups about potential cancer-causing properties of propyl gallate.

Sodium Benzoate:

1. This preservative is derived from benzoic acid, which occurs naturally in many foods.

2. Sodium benzoate is used to prevent the growth of bacteria and other microorganisms, but is effective only when added to foods and drinks that are highly acidic, such as fruit juices, carbonated drinks, and pickles

3. The FDA considers sodium benzoate to be safe, although some people are allergic to it.

Sodium Nitrite:

1. This preservative is the salt of nitrous acid.

2. Sodium nitrite is used as a preservative in bacon, ham, hotdogs, and most cold cuts.

3. This additive may cause cancer, but the Department of Agriculture claims it is required in order to prevent botulism.

Sorbic Acid:

1. This preservative occurs naturally in the berries of the mountain ash and in a number of plants.

2. Sorbic acid is used to prevent the growth of molds and fungi in foods and beverages such as cheese, mayonnaise, jelly, margarine, wine, and soft drinks.

3. This additive appears to be safe.

Sulfiting Agents:

1. This preservative includes sulfur dioxide, sodium bisulfite, and sodium sulfite compounds.

2. Sulfiting agents are used to retard the growth of bacteria and to prevent the discoloration of foods such as:

    a. Canned meat

    b. Dried foods

    c. Maraschino cherries

    d. Wines, beers, and some fruit drinks

    e. Lettuce and other raw vegetables served at salad bars

    f. Dried foods

    g. Seafood (especially shrimp)

    h. Dips, especially those with avocado

    i. Some asthma medications, including Alupent®, Bronkosol®, and Isuprel®.

3. Between 1 and 5% of asthmatic patients are allergic to sulfites, which are the only additives in use known to have caused fatal allergic reactions. At the prompting of the FDA, most processors now include a warning on their label that states that the food includes sulfites.

EMULSIFIERS

These are substances that enable oil and water to mix.

Lecithin:

1. This emulsifier is found in most plant and animal tissues.

2. Lecithin is used as a food additive.

3. Lecithin is a good source of choline, one of the B vitamins.

Monoglycerides & Diglycerides:

1. These emulsifiers are metabolized by the body in a manner similar to fat.

2. The additives are found in chocolate, bread, margarine, cake, and peanut butter.

3. Monoglycerides and diglycerides are safe but diminish the nutritional value of some foods.

Polysorbates 60, 65, & 80:

1. These emulsifiers are made from the reaction of fatty acids with sorbitol.

2. The additives prevent flavor oils like vanilla, strawberry, and lemon from separating out of ice cream, beverages, and candy.

3. There is some concern among FDA scientists as to whether or not the levels of polysorbates in foods are too high.

THICKENERS & STABILIZERS

Thickening agents add body to foods and improve their texture and consistency.

Carboxymethylcellulose:

1. Carboxymethylcellulose is a derivative of cellulose.

2. The additive is used as a thickener and stabilizer in ice cream, beer, jelly, cake icing, and other foods and beverages. It is also added to diet foods.

3. Carboxymethylcellulose is considered safe in limited quantities.

Carrageenan:

1. This thickener is extracted from the seaweed Irish Moss.

2. It is added to many processed milk products.

3. Carrageenans are fine for adults, but could inhibit the development of the gastrointestinal tract of premature infants.

Locus Bean Gum:

1. Locus bean gum comes from the bean of the carob tree.

2. The additive is used in salad dressings, barbecue sauce, and other foods.

3. Locus bean gum is considered to be safe in small quantities.

Modified Starches:

1. These thickeners are produced by the breakdown of natural starch.

2. They are used in many sauces and to prevent sugar from crystallizing in candy.

3. The additive can displace more nutritious ingredients.

Sodium Alginate:

1. Sodium alginate is created by the reaction of sodium and alginic acid, a sugar found in giant kelp and other forms of seaweed.

2. It is added to a wide range of foods, including ice cream, canned frosting, cheese, candy, condiments, and relish.

3. In large quantities, sodium alginate may interfere with vitamin and mineral absorption.

FLAVOR ENHANCERS

These are chemicals added to food to enhance their natural taste.

Disodium Guanylate (GMP):

1. This enhancer is found in certain mushrooms and some species of fish.

2. GMP is added to many soup mixes, sandwich spreads, and canned vegetables..

3. The body converts GMP to uric acid. If you have a tendency towards gout, this could be a problem.

Monosodium Glutamate (MSG):

1. MSG is derived from glutamic acid, one of the amino acids.

2. MSG heightens the flavor of foods such as canned soup, bouillon cubes, cheese, and processed meats.

3. MSG is thought to be the cause of "Chinese restaurant syndrome," the symptoms of which include headaches and tightening of the muscles of the face, neck, and chest.

OTHER ADDITIVES

Tartrazine (Yellow Food Dye #5):

1. This additive can affect aspirin-sensitive patients.

2. Tartrazine is added to:

   a. yellow cake mixes;   c. beverages; and

   b. some candies;   d. some medications.

REDUCING CHEMICALS AND IRRITANTS FROM THE HOME (adapted from Gilbert, 1987).

The following irritants or allergens should be removed from the homes of patients with asthma (Gilbert, 1987):

ASBESTOS:

This fibrous mineral has been used to insulate walls and heating pipes, to soundproof rooms, to fireproof walls and fireplaces, to strengthen vinyl floors and joint compounds, and to provide paint with texture.

Asbestos poses a health hazard only if fibers are released into the air. In remodeling homes constructed between 1920 and 1970, this can occur. Inhaled fibers can cause (a) cancer of the lung, stomach, and chest lining; and (b) asbestosis, a lung disease that is usually fatal. Asbestos and smoking are a particularly deadly combination.

RADON:

This radioactive gas is the second leading cause of lung cancer in the U.S. (behind cigarette smoking). When you breathe in radon, it becomes trapped in your lungs and assaults them with radiation. Radon is produced by the decay of uranium in soil and rocks. It does not appear to be an outdoor health hazard; it becomes a problem only when it accumulates in an enclosed area. Radon enters the house through drainpipes or cracks in foundations and concrete basement walls.

Local health departments, as well as the American Lung Association, have published a number of free booklets on radon gas for those who may suspect it is entering their homes. They explain the tests that can be conducted to detect the gas.

FORMALDEHYDE:

It is almost impossible to avoid formaldehyde gas: Formaldehyde is in everything from wood paneling to toothpaste. Formaldehyde has been used in construction and manufacturing for the past 100 years; fumes from the product can cause chronic respiratory problems, dizziness, rashes, lethargy, and nausea.

The 3-M Corporation makes an inexpensive device (approximately $50) that can be put into the home to assess whether the amount of formaldehyde exceeds Federal standards as to what is a safe environment. A method for removing formaldehyde from the home is to buy a number of house plants. According to experts, 15 to 20 plants would remove the formaldehyde from an 1,800 square foot home.

WATER POLLUTION:

It is estimated that 2% of the country's community water supplies pose a significant risk to our health. About 38 million Americans are estimated to drink water tainted with unsafe levels of lead. This can lead to hypertension in adults, learning disabilities in children, neurological damage in fetuses, and miscarriages. The best way to correct this problem is to contact your local water supplier. In addition, the EPA recommends running your cold water for approximately 2 minutes each morning to flush out water that has been sitting in the pipes all night, thus accumulating lead.

HOUSEHOLD CHEMICALS:

Many of the products we use to clean, beautify, and fumigate our homes and gardens can also cause serious illnesses. These chemicals have been linked to cancer and respiratory ailments, as well as nausea and dizziness. Ammonia, for example, can inflame the respiratory tract and serve as a trigger of attacks in some asthmatic patients.

Pesticides on the market--there are 50,000 different products to choose from--have been linked to cancer and reproductive problems.

Two ways have been suggested to eliminate the effect of household chemicals as a cause of respiratory distress: (1) use safer alternatives, such as water-based paints, beeswax floor cleaners, etc., and (2) always ventilate the home well when painting, or using paint thinners or cleaners. Store these materials outdoors; otherwise, they will dry out and the vapors will escape into your home.

COMBUSTION GASES:

Any appliance that burns fuel discharges combustion gases such as carbon dioxide. If these gases build up in your home, they can trigger asthma attacks and cause chronic bronchitis, headaches, dizziness, nausea, and fatigue. Wood-burning stoves discharge smoke that can also trigger attacks.

To prevent these gases from causing health problems, the best solution is to be certain they are serviced regularly and placed in well-ventilated areas of the house.

ALLERGENS:

One out of every six Americans is allergic to something. There are a number of air-cleaning products on the market that can sometimes help reduce the amount of air pollution in the home. Other suggestions include:

1. Thoroughly cleaning your home on a regular basis;

2. Clean humidifiers and drain dehumidifiers once a week so that allergens and mold are not continually disseminated throughout your home;

3. Service air-conditioning units and clean their filters every spring;

4. Keep clean filters in your furnace; and

5. Rid your home of any pets that may give off animal dander and trigger your asthma. Despite the old-wives tale that it is the length of the animal's hair that is the culprit in triggering asthma, it should be pointed out that the dander from any animal with hair can precipitate attacks.

WAYS TO MANAGE A COMMON COLD WITH THE AIM OF PREVENTING ASTHMA ATTACKS (suggested by M. Castleman, 1987).

1. **Rest.** Since it takes effort to fight a cold, the patient should obtain all the rest he or she can. The patient should take it easy. It may prevent either an exacerbation of the cold or prevent an asthma flare-up.

2. **Bundle up.** This helps alleviate those colds that are accompanied by fever.

3. **Stop smoking.** If the patient hasn't stopped smoking because of asthma, a cold will offer you the perfect opportunity to finally bounce the poisonous weed from daily life.

4. **Drink eight ounces of warm liquids every two hours.** This procedure will not only soothe a sore throat and relieve nasal congestion, but it will prevent the patient from becoming dehydrated. The latter may be of value in the event the patient later suffers an asthma attack.

5. **For sore throat, gargle with warm salt water, suck on hard candies, and increase relative humidity.** Castleman (1987) notes that the recommended salt mixture is one-half teaspoon per eight ounces. An occasional hot shower can help humidify lungs and environment.

6. **For fever, headaches, and body aches, try a cool cloth on the forehead or use a medication, such as acetaminophen or ibuprofen, that has been recommended by a physician.**

7. **For nasal congestion, drink warm fluids, or use a vaporizer, hot bath, or shower. At night, use extra pillows to elevate the head.** If the patient has a cold, he or she may wish to contact a physician. The physician can advise on the proper use and care of a vaporizer. It is important that the physician's advice be followed, as misuse of a vaporizer can create problems for asthmatic patients.

8. **Use disposable tissues.** Besides following this advice, always wash hands after blowing the nose. This practice helps prevent the virus from passing along to other family members. The patient should always clean any glass from which he or she has drunk liquids; do not leave it on a counter for other family members to use.

9. **Do not suppress productive coughs.** It is always helpful to cough up the mucous and other substances that accumulate in the throat and lungs.

10. **Antibiotics are useless against colds.** These compounds are excellent against bacterial infections, but they are useless against viral infections. In addition, there is the possibility that such medications can interact in a negative manner with asthma drugs.

11. **Avoid time-release medications.** While convenient, they fall short of their claims. The patient should ask a physician about any cold medications he or she is considering before taking them.

12. **Remember some of grandma's methods of dealing with a cold.** There seems to be evidence that hot chicken soup and other remedies suggested by grandmothers have some role in the treatment of a viral infection. They are worth a try.

SAFE USE OF MEDICATIONS

IMPORTANT INFORMATION FOR INTERACTING WITH PHYSICIANS

A.   **Provide medical history.** The patient should tell the important facts of his or her history with medicines. Any allergic reactions experienced, any side-effects, or any other adverse effects attributed to the medications should be described. The patient should be precise in describing allergic reactions such as asthma attacks, hay fever, watery eyes and itching, or throat irritation. Allergic individuals are more apt to experience these types of reactions than are those with no known allergies.

B.   **Medicines now being taken by patient.** The patient should be certain to mention all prescription and non-prescription drugs. The latter include such commonly used medicines as:

   a. laxatives

   b. vitamin or mineral supplements

   c. skin, rectal, or vaginal medicines

   d. antacids or antigas medicines

   e. antihistamines

   f. cold and cough remedies

   g. aspirin and medicines that contain aspirin

   h. motion sickness medicines

   i. weight-loss aids

   j. salt and sugar substitutes

   k. caffeine products

   l. oral contraceptives

   m. sleeping pills

   n. tonics

INFORMATION A PATIENT SHOULD KNOW BEFORE OR IN TAKING ANY ASTHMA MEDICINE

1. The generic names and brand names of all medicines taken. The patient should jot them down to help remember. If a medicine is a mixture of two or more generic ingredients, he or she should know the names of each.

   a. Patient should write down all medication instructions and never rely on memory.

2. The uses of each medicine taken.

3. The best way to fit a medicine into a patient's regular routine.

4. The dose and schedule of each medicine.

   a. Reduce the number of times a medication is taken daily if possible.

5. What the patient should do if he or she forgets to take a dose of medicine.

6. How each medicine works in the body.

7. The time lapse that can be expected before a drug begins to take action.

8. The symptoms and treatment of an overdose of a medicine.

9. Possible side-effects and adverse reactions that might be experienced and what to do when they occur.

10. Periodically review all medications with physician to see if any can be dropped from regimen.

11. The interactions of any given medicine with other drugs, alcohol, beverages, foods, cocaine, marijuana, and tobacco. The interaction of many of these compounds can often lead to life-threatening situations.

12. The patient should know all the warnings and precautions that apply to special circumstances such as:

    a. Reasons for not taking drug in the presence of some medical condition. These reasons are called contraindications; a good example for many asthmatic patients is to avoid aspirin even if they are experiencing a headache.

    b. Special considerations for children, elderly patients, or pregnant or breast-feeding women.

    c. Such factors as any implications of prolonged use, effects resulting from exposure to sun and sunlight, and any changes that can affect driving, hazardous work, or flying in airplanes.

    d. Any instructions that must be considered before discontinuing a drug. A prime illustration would be suggestions for reducing steroid preparations taken to help control asthma.

OTHER TIPS

1. Before any elective surgery and during pregnancy or breast-feeding, the patient should discuss the use of medicines with a physician.

2. The patient should not hesitate to ask a physician questions about a particular drug. It is better that the physician provide answers for the patient than for the patient to suffer in ignorance.

3. The patient should never take medicine in the dark. It is always possible to take the wrong drug; the label should always be rechecked before each drug use.

4. The patient should be certain to explain to the physician about any new or unexpected symptoms developed while taking medicine. The physician may wish either to adjust the amount of medicine taken or change drugs.

5. All medications should be kept out of the reach of children and others. Medicines should be kept in a cool, dry place such as a kitchen cabinet or bedroom. The patient should avoid keeping medicine in bathrooms as they may become too moist or warm. Medicines should be kept in the original container and tightly closed. Labels should never be removed!

6. Leftover oral or injectable medicine should never be saved for later use. It should be discarded before or on the expiration date displayed on the container. Any leftover medicine should be disposed of so as to protect children and pets.

7. The patient should study any information, particularly drug inserts. If there are any questions about a drug, the patient should write them down and ask the physician during the next visit.

8. Medicine that has been prescribed for someone else should never be taken; it could interact with prescribed drugs presently that are being taken by the patient.

9. Prior to any surgery, including any dental procedures, the patient should be certain to inform the physician or dentist about all medicines being taken or that have been taken in the past few weeks. The anesthesiologist would like to know the patient has asthma in case something occurs during surgery.

10. The patient should carefully evaluate any generic medicine received. Not all generic drugs are as effective as other asthma drugs; if the patient believes such medicines are not as effective as brand-name products, he or she should be certain to inform the physician of this opinion and belief.

11. The patient with allergies should review his or her medication needs before a season occurs when the patient is apt to suffer more attacks.

12. The patient should keep abreast of the introduction of any new asthma medications that come onto the market. He or she may then wish to discuss these preparations with his or her physician.

References

Ballard, R. D., & Martin, R. J. (1987). Nocturnal asthma. Seminars in Respiratory Medicine, 8, 302-307.

Castleman, M. (1987). Cold Cures. New York: Fawcett Columbine.

Creer, T. L. (1983). Response: Self-management psychology and the treatment of childhood asthma. Journal of Allergy & Clinical Immunology, 72, 607-610.

Gilbert, S. (September 27, 1987). Home remedies: A sensible approach to finding and eliminating indoor pollutants. New York Times Magazine, Part 2, 26-27, 36-37, 40.

Griffith, H. W. (1985). Complete guide to symptoms, illness, and surgery. Los Angeles, CA: The Body Press.

Kaliner, M., Eggleston, P.A., & Mathews, K.P. (1987). Rhinitis and asthma. JAMA, 258, 2851-2873.

Kanfer, F. H. (1980). Self-management methods. In F. H. Kanfer & A. P. (Eds.), Helping People Change. Second edition. New York: Pergamon Press, 334-389.

Klockenbrink, M. (September 27,1987). How to read a label. New York Times Magazine, Part 2, 67-68, 72.

Marion, R. J. (1987). Teaching children to predict asthma using an in-home pulmometer. Unpublished doctoral dissertation, Ohio University, Athens, Ohio.

Martin, G., & Pear, J. (1988). Behavior modification: What it is and how to use it. Englewood Cliffs, NJ: Prentice-Hall.

O'Leary, S. G., & Dubey, D. R. (1979). Applications of self-control procedures by children: A review. Journal of Applied Behavior Analysis, 12, 449-465.

Sampson, H.A., Buckley, R.H., & Metcalfe, D.D. (1987). Food allergy. JAMA, 258, 2886-2890.

Simon, R. A. (1984). Environmental control and dust abatement. In A. Dawson & R. A. Simon (Eds.), The practical management of asthma. Orlando: Grune & Stratton.

Watson, D. L., & Tharp, R. G. (1989). Self-directed behavior: Self-modification for personal adjustment. Fifth edition. Monterey, CA: Brooks/Cole Publishing Company.

MEDICATION COMPLIANCE
VISUAL 3.1

REASONS FOR NONCOMPLIANCE	SOLUTIONS
Expense (medications and office visits)	Shop around; do not buy inhaler dispenser each time; let physician know money is a concern to you; consider SSI; ask doctor to call in order; have several refills on each medication
Taste	Take medicine with foods or beverage if appropriate
Inconvenient schedule	Ask physician to change schedule to fit a routine; you may request a time released preparation
Absent or undetectable asthma symptoms	Remind yourself that asthma is a variable and intermittent disorder; always consult with physician about stopping medications
Asthma symptoms while on medications	Talk with your physician; a change in medications may be in order
Unclear instructions	Ask physician or pharmacist to clarify directions
Social stigma	Educate family and friends about asthma and the need for medications

<u>MEDICATION COMPLIANCE</u>
VISUAL 3.1 (contd.)

REASONS FOR NONCOMPLIANCE	SOLUTIONS
Side effects	Learn about medication side effects; report side effects to physician; your doctor may prescribe different dose levels, forms, or types of medication
Poor relationship with physician	Be active; change physician if questions go repeatedly unanswered

<u>ASTHMA TRIGGERS</u>
VISUAL 3.2

<u>TRIGGER</u>	<u>COPING STRATEGIES</u>
Stress (emotional, behavioral, and cognitive responses to situations)	Identify and avoid stressful situations, use stress-management skills (relaxation, exercise)
Exercise	Be alert to early warning signs; slowly increase the intensity and duration of exercise
Mechanical triggers (sneezing, coughing laughing, crying, and choking)	Treat congestion and post nasal drip; use relaxation to avoid strong emotional responses
Respiratory infections	Follow good health practice; obtain regular flu shots, treat colds and infections early
Allergens/Pollen	Minimize outdoor activities during allergy seasons; obtain allergy injections
Dust, animal dander, molds	Keep house clean; use polyester materials (pillows, rugs, curtains, bedding); use plastic mattress covers; use rubber rug/carpet pads; avoid contact with pets
Foods and food additives (mold, sodium benzoate, sulfates, monosodium glutamate, yellow dye)	Avoid trigger foods; refrigerate foods as soon as opened and used; read labels

ASTHMA TRIGGERS
VISUAL 3.2 (contd.)

TRIGGER	COPING STRATEGIES
Irritants (cigarette smoke, formaldehyde, household cleaners, combustion gases)	Quit smoking; limit others smoking indoors; wear air filter mask; keep indoor plants; avoid toxic cleaners; store toxic liquids outdoors; have wood burning stoves and furnaces serviced frequently and placed in well-ventilated areas
Air pollutants (sulfur dioxide, ozone, nitrogen dioxide)	Monitor outside air quality daily, live away from heavy manufacturing; avoid rush hour exposure; do not burn trash or lawn debris
Cold Air	Dress appropriately; wear scarf over mouth; avoid exercise outdoors in cold, dry weather

ASTHMA EARLY WARNING SIGNS

VISUAL 3.3

Common Physical Early Warning Signs

Very common
Coughing
Shortness of breath
Tightness in chest
Chest hurts
Decreased exercise tolerance
Chest filling up
Taking deep breaths
Breathing through the mouth

Common
Feeling tired
Headache
Itchy, sore, scratchy throat
Watery eyes
Feverish
Dry mouth
Clammy skin, increased
    sweating
Pale facial color
Swollen face
Flared nostrils
Bad breath
Heart beating faster
Sneezing
Congestion
Dark circles under the eyes
Quickening breathing

Common Emotional Early Warning Signs

Difficulty concentrating
Getting upset easily
Feeling nervous
Feeling sad, down
Getting excited easily
Feeling grumpy
Wanting to be alone
Feeling restless
Becoming quiet
Feeling tired, fatigued

SOLVED PROBLEMS EXERCISE
VISUAL 3.4

(1) $\underline{S}$tate the problem.	
(2) $\underline{O}$utline the problem.	
(3)$\underline{L}$ist solutions. a.	(4)$\underline{V}$iew the consequences. +
	-
b.	+
	-
c.	+
	-
d.	+
	-
e.	+
	-
f.	+
	-
(5)$\underline{E}$xecute your solution.	
(6)$\underline{D}$etermine if solution is effective.	

SESSION FOUR
MANAGING ATTACKS

GOALS
1. Describe signs of worsening asthma.
2. Describe signs of severe asthma.
3. Review asthma self-management steps:
   a. Rest and relax (practice relaxation in session).
   b. Drink warm liquids.
   c. Use medicines prescribed for attacks.
   d. Contact family member or friend.
   e. Call physician.

EQUIPMENT
Name tags.
Recliner chairs or pillows and mats for the floor.
Paper and pencils for all participants.
Overhead projector or slide projector.
Relaxation tapes for each subject.

SUPPLIES
Coffee, tea, snacks, or light lunch.

SESSION FOUR OUTLINE

TOPIC/ ACTIVITY	REQUIRED MATERIAL	APPROXIMATE TIME ALLOWED
Welcome & salutations	Name tags	5 minutes
Questions about prior sessions/readings		10 minutes
Signs of worsening asthma	Visual 4.1	10 minutes
Signs of severe asthma	Visual 4.2	10 minutes
Asthma self-management steps	Visual 4.3	20 minutes
1) Relaxation: Deep breathing/ Deep muscle relaxation	Visual 4.4, 4.5	
2) Drink warm liquids	Visual 4.6	
3) Medications for attacks	Visual 4.7	
4) Contact family & friends for support	Visual 4.8	
5) Call a physician/ emergency medical services	Visual 4.9	
Practice relaxation	Reclining chairs or bedrolls and pillows	20 minutes
Open discussion		15 minutes
Homework	Practice relaxation twice daily, read Chapter 6	5 minutes

SESSION FOUR TEACHING NOTES

Welcome and Salutations

Provide a name tag for each participant. Allow time for small talk among group members prior to introducing the session.

Questions About Prior Sessions/Readings

Allow the group time to ask questions about material covered earlier in the program.

Signs of Worsening Asthma

Rely on the group to report their own experience of worsening asthma before introducing the complete list with Visual 4.1. Help the group distinguish between early warning signs and signs of worsening asthma.

Signs of Severe Asthma

Let the group relate their own experience of severe asthma signs and when they think it necessary to seek medical help. Introduce Visual 4.2 and discuss the decision to seek medical help. Help the group distinguish between early warning signs, signs of worsening asthma, and signs of severe asthma.

Self-Management Steps

Stress that the best time to treat an attack is when early warning signs appear. Provide an overview of the rationale of self-management--it is a step-by-step problem-solving approach. Self-care strategies are arranged in a hierarchy; self-management behaviors at each step are usually tried before going on to other steps. Encourage discussion by eliciting management steps the group has found helpful before presenting Visual 4.3.

1. **Deep Breathing and Deep Muscle Relaxation Exercise.** Introduce relaxation techniques, discussing the use of deep breathing, deep muscle relaxation, and imagery. Encourage clients to use any method of relaxation they have found effective in the past, such as meditation, yoga, or prayer. Relaxation can produce direct improvement in lung functioning, and offers a proven method of controlling anxiety reactions associated with asthma episodes. In addition to preventing mild attacks, use of relaxation can help one maintain a problem-solving attitude when managing more severe attacks. (See Visuals 4.4, 4.5.)

2. **Drinking Warm Liquids.** Review the rationale behind drinking warm liquids during an attack, discuss the need for rehydration, and discuss the bronchodilation effects of warm liquids. (See Visual 4.6.)

3. **Use of Prescribed Medicines During Attacks.** Discuss the types of medications that should be used during an attack, and the types of drugs that might exacerbate the attack or have no effect. Let the group discuss how long they think they should wait before taking more medications or calling the physician if the medications are not working. (See Visual 4.7.)

4. **Use of Family & Friends for Support.** Ask the group to brainstorm about natural support systems they have available to them. Discuss who can help them manage and cope with attacks. (See Visual 4.8.)

5. **Call a Physician/Emergency Medical Services.** Encourage the group to discuss how they feel about calling a physician during a severe attack--do they feel reluctant to call? Review the signs of severe asthma. (See Visual 4.9.)

Relaxation Exercise

Lead the group through the deep breathing and deep muscle relaxation exercises. Make sure that everyone is in a comfortable position, ideally in recliner chairs or using pillows and mats on the floor. Allow at least 20 minutes for the exercise.

Open Discussion

Allow time for a general question and answer period. Encourage the group to answer each other's questions where possible.

Homework

Encourage participants to practice deep breathing and deep muscle relaxation one or two times per day during the week. Emphasize the need for practice, and explain that these techniques do not work like medications, i.e., that they can't expect them to work immediately. Practice is necessary in order for the techniques to be effective. Advise the clients to read Chapter 6 before next session.

SESSION FOUR BACKGROUND READING

ARTERIAL BLOOD GAS ABNORMALITIES THAT OCCUR WITH INCREASING SEVERITY OF ASTHMA ATTACKS

ATTACK SEVERITY	ARTERIAL OXYGEN PRESSURE	ARTERIAL CARBON DIOXIDE PRESSURE	pH
MILD	Normal	Slight decrease	Slight elevation
MODERATE	Slight decrease	Slight decrease	Slight elevation
SEVERE	Moderate decrease	Normal	Normal
VERY SEVERE	Substantial decrease	Slight to moderate increase	Decrease

ANAPHYLACTIC REACTION

There are times when a person is exposed to a stimulus and an immediate hypersensitivity reaction occurs. The stimulus could be an allergen, an insect sting or, in some occasions, the rapid inhalation of too much cold, dry air. The reaction that comprises anaphylaxis is characterized by abdominal cramps, diarrhea, dizziness, and weakness. Difficulty in breathing, a rapid drop in blood pressure, and unconsciousness may also occur.

Immediate medical attention is required with anaphylactic reactions. When help is not immediately available, such as to the person who may be stung by an insect when in a wilderness area, a self-administered injection of adrenaline is necessary. A physician will inform the patient if he or she is at risk for an anaphylactic reaction. The physician may immunize the patient if insect bites are apt to trigger such reactions; if this does not seem a workable solution, the physician may ask the patient to carry a kit with adrenalin.

THE ABCDs OF TREATING AN ASTHMA ATTACK
(Adapted from Winder, 1984)

A - ACTIVITY & ATTITUDE ADJUSTMENT

THINK OF THE THREE Rs:

REST--Stop all activity and rest.
RELAX--Settle down and think about how previous attacks have been managed.
RIGHT BREATHING--Purse lips as if to whistle and exhale slowly. Then inhale normally. Repeat this several times.

If A does not bring about relief from the attack within 3 to 5 minutes, go on to Step B.

B - BRONCHODILATORS

Use whatever inhaled bronchodilator has been prescribed by your physician. By following proper instructions for use of the bronchodilator, bronchospasms should relax and the airways should open.

Once Step B has been completed, go on to Step C.

C - CONSUME LIQUIDS

Drink 12 to 32 ounces of room-temperature to lukewarm clear liquid--water, juice, soft drink--over a 15 to 30 minute period. This will thin the mucus so that it can be coughed out for easier breathing. It will also provide a self-management skill for you to perform.

D - CALL THE DOC

The patient should call his or her doctor for further instructions under the following conditions:

1. When Steps A, B, and C do not diminish the attack within 2 hours, the process should be repeated. If the patient has to use A, B, and C three times in any 24-hour period, the physician should be called. Remember that ABC x 3 = D.

2. When wheezing seems to worsen after there has been time for the inhaled medication to work. This is particularly important when the patient has used the nebulizer twice within a short period of time.

3. When, even with pursed-lips breathing, wheezing continues.

4. When shoulders are hunched, it is difficult to talk or move, it feels as though breathing can only be done from the neck up, nostrils are flared, or lips or nails are beginning to turn blue.

5. When 30 or more breaths per minute are taken.

6. When there are questions about what to do. Remember that ET means earlier treatment: the sooner the patient controls asthma, the earlier it is to control.

RELAXATION PROCEDURES

In addition to the deep muscle relaxation training stressed throughout this program, there are other relaxation techniques that can be used by patients with asthma. Some patients, if they are skilled at performing these techniques, may wish to use them in place of deep muscle relaxation. Most patients, however, will be unfamiliar with any type of relaxation procedure; for them, deep muscle relaxation should be the method of choice. If there are individual patients who appear to require additional training, components of other procedures may be added to their training. The procedures to be briefly described are: (1) autogenic training; (2) meditation; and (3) systematic desensitization.

AUTOGENIC TRAINING

This method originated in Europe at the turn of the century from the sleep and hypnosis research of Oskar Vogt in Berlin (Schultz & Luthe, 1959). Yoga was added as an ingredient in the training. Basically, autogenic therapy consists of a series of six standard exercises aimed at relaxing both the mind and the body. The six are: (a) heaviness; (b) warmth; (c) cardiac regulation; (d) respiration; (e) abdominal warmth; and (f) cooling of the forehead. Only heaviness and warmth, however, are exercises used in the United States. The exercises are employed in the following manner:

First, patients are instructed to relax in a quiet room and in a comfortable position. Here, the procedure is identical to that followed with deep muscle relaxation. A point stressed in autogenic training is that the exercises be conducted with an attitude of passive concentration.

Second, when patients are told to tighten the muscles of their dominant arm, they are also told to imagine that an "arm is heavy." This phrase is repeated in much the same manner as that used with deep muscle relaxation.

Third, this procedure is repeated, usually over the course of several days. According to Rudestam:

> "It will probably take several days of training with the dominant arm before you experience a distinct, heavy feeling there. Don't try to force the heaviness; passively allow it to build. When the heaviness occurs reliably, do the exercise with your other arm, proceeding in exactly the same way. Once you have experienced a distinct heavy feeling in the nondominant arm as well, repeat the exercise for both arms for several days then turn to the dominant leg. Say to yourself, 'my right (left) leg is heavy,' then gradually move on to 'My left (right) leg is heavy,' and eventually suggest, 'Both legs are heavy.' Don't rush yourself. After many practice sessions, you will be ready for the summary statement: 'My arms and legs are heavy'" (1980, p. 29).

Finally, when the feelings of heaviness in the patient's arms and legs occur quickly, the feeling supposedly generalizes from the limbs to the patient's entire body. When this occurs, it is time to move on to the second autogenic exercise, the encouragement of warmth. The patient is instructed, in a manner similar to that described above, to imagine he or she is experiencing sensations of warmth in his or her limbs. Again, the patient is asked to practice the procedure for several days until he or she spontaneously experiences the feelings of warmth.

Self-induced states of heaviness and warmth are a good means of relaxing by controlling bodily sensations. Schultz and Luthe (1959) reported that autogenic training was useful with a variety of physical disorders, including asthma.

MEDITATION

In the past decades, considerable interest has been shown in the United States with respect to a number of Eastern approaches to relaxation. Chief among what are regarded as meditation techniques are Yoga meditation, Zen meditation, and, in particular, Transcendental Meditation. All are based on the notion that we can shift our attention away from ongoing concerns toward the exercise being performed. Exclusive attention is paid to the meditation object, which may range from focusing entirely upon your breathing to the repeated recitation of a mantra, a melodic phrase or word. The differences in these techniques are sometimes subtle:

1. **Transcendental Meditation (TM).** This consists of the repetition of a mantra twice a day for about twenty minutes. The mantra, a word such as "Om" or "Da-Mi," has no English meaning. Nevertheless, by repeating the word, one can begin to passively let go of thoughts and associations. Rudestam (1980) describes the following Transcendental Meditation exercise:

> "Assume a comfortable position. Concentrate continuously on your sound, repeating it subvocally, slowly and rhythmically over and over. If your concentration wanders, as it is bound to, gently return to the mantra, repeating it over and over. Perhaps the most significant aspect of the meditation procedure is that you do not work at concentrating on your mantra; instead you adopt a passive attitude and allow the thoughts in your consciousness to move on past you. Let whatever happens happen. If memories, preoccupations, or mental images appear, observe them with detachment, let them slide by, and return to silently repeating your mantra. At first the mantra may mean something to you. After a while you stop thinking of the meaning and get involved with the sound. Eventually the meaning disappears completely and the sound becomes totally compelling and achieves a vibrancy of its own" (p. 33).

Those who practice TM believe that it is a learned skill; however, they caution, it must be practiced daily in order to reap the benefits of the procedure.

2. **Yoga meditation.** Rudestam (1980) points out that those who practice Yoga believe three different disciplines are involved: (a) the ethico-religious discipline is a set of rules for conduct which are designed to maintain mental and physical purity; (b) the physical-vital discipline consists of eating a well-balanced diet, maintaining close ties to nature, and being kind to the body; and (c) the psycho-spiritual discipline entails withdrawing attention from the outside world and rechanneling energy to one specific focus or direction.

The form of yoga meditation that consists of bringing your mind to one focal point is called vipassana. The purpose of vipassana is to experience objects as they are. Rudestam (1980) notes that sensory stimuli are supposed to receive scant attention; sensory perceptions are simply noticed and not allowed to stimulate chain reactions of thought. He describes an exercise that can be practiced to attain this state:

> "Try to focus on the tip of your nose and note your breath going in and out for 15 seconds. Just notice the breath at the tip of the nose, not when it moves into your body or when it drifts into space" (p. 35).

Detachment from the senses is important to the meditative process. There are several ways this aim can be achieved; most involve concentrating on an unchanged visual stimulus. This may be anything from a vase to specifically prepared designs called mandalas. The latter are circular motifs in which all lines converge in the center. In meditating on a mandala, your attention is drawn to the inner circle, the center of the mandala where consciousness changes. The design, suggests Rudestam (1980), is intended to induce total mental calm and the feeling of being centered. In another form of Yoga, called pranayama, attention is focused on the breathing cycle. Changes in oxygen intake and use lead to physiological changes and, in some cases, to changes in awareness.

3. **Zen meditation.** Rudestam (1980) describes what he refers to as a well-known Zen meditation and breathing exercise:

> "Assume a comfortable position and breathe through your nose. Count each time you exhale, from one to ten, and then count back again from ten to one. As you begin to pay attention to your breathing, you may initially experience a sensation of breathing shallowly and of not getting enough air. This difficulty will pass as you repeat the process of counting to ten and back with your exhalations. You may have difficulty focusing on the breaths and be distracted by irrelevant thoughts and images. If this happens, merely note that your attention has wandered. Do not follow the thoughts; relax and return to the task of breathing. Gradually the task will become 'effortless' and you will be able to focus on breathing while concomitantly observing the fears, thoughts, fantasies, and events that are competing for your attention. In time these thoughts may become less disturbing and intrusive, and eventually, they may drift away completely" (p. 37).

The use of a Zen breathing exercise, very similar to those performed in deep muscle relaxation, is often combined with use of a mantra to form a complete meditation practice.

In his popular book, Benson (1975) suggested a method of relaxation that is based upon meditation. He includes the following steps which are similar to those taught patients in the Client's Guide:

a. Once or twice a day, find a quiet place. Sit comfortably and close your eyes.

b. Practice the deep muscle relaxation skills you have been taught. Try and keep yourself relaxed.

c. Become aware of your breathing by breathing naturally through your nose. As you exhale, silently say to yourself a word such as "om" or even "one."

d. Maintain a passive attitude. Let relaxation come to you. If distracting thoughts enter your consciousness, try not to dwell upon them.

e. Finally, practice the exercise for 10 to 20 minutes. You may look at a clock to check the time, but avoid the use of an alarm clock. When you finish, sit quietly with your eyes closed for a few minutes. You are then asked to open your eyes and sit still for a few more minutes before you stand.

SYSTEMATIC DESENSITIZATION

Systematic desensitization is perhaps the most widely used behavioral therapy technique. It is included here because it has been found useful in the management of asthma (Miklich, Renne, Creer, Alexander, Chai, Davis, Hoffman, & Danker-Brown, 1977). The procedure involves three separate stages:

1. Patients are initially taught to relax via deep muscle relaxation training. After these skills have been mastered by the patient, he or she can move to the next stage of systematic desensitization.

2. Patients are asked to briefly describe situations that particularly cause them to experience emotional distress. These should center on stimuli surrounding their asthma, such as fear that an attack will intensify, that they may not be able to breathe, or that they may need treatment at a hospital emergency room. The instructor should review these descriptions with a patient to be certain that all aspects of the fear-provoking situation are reported by the patient. When the instructor believes he or she has elicited all of this information from the patient, the instructor and patient can arrange the fear-evoking stimuli into a hierarchy of items that revolve around a common theme. Depending upon the material presented by the patient, the instructor may compose a hierarchy of 5 to 15 items, extending from the least fearful to the most fearful aspect of the situation. It can be expected that anywhere from 3 to 8 hierarchies will be presented by any given patient. These can include themes ranging from fears of suffering an attack to specific experiences that comprise an asthmatic episode. Many patients provide information on the settings where attacks occur; this information, too, can be transposed into a hierarchy by the instructor.

3. The final and most crucial stage of systematic desensitization is to pair deep muscle relaxation with items presented from the hierarchies. This is the desensitization phase of the technique. After patients are relaxed, they are asked to imagine a situation or setting in which they find pleasure. This may be anything from resting beside the banks of a slow-moving stream on a warm summer day to viewing their favorite television program. When patients have this scene clearly in mind, they should signal their perception to the instructor. If patients are practicing this procedure by themselves, they should move on to the next stage of systematic desensitization. The next stage entails that the item from a hierarchy that arouses the least amount of fear or anxiety be imagined by the patient. If he or she can imagine this scene and still remain relaxed, the patient is instructed to imagine the next item on the hierarchy, moving from items that induce the least amount of anxiety to the items that elicit the greatest amount of anxiety. If the patient can remain relaxed while moving up the hierarchy, he or she is asked to continue the desensitization process. If, however, the patient begins to feel anxious or fearful, he or she is asked to imagine either the neutral scene or an item on the hierarchy that no longer elicits anxiety or fear. When they have demonstrated to themselves that they have desensitized themselves to stimuli that formerly elicited emotional reactions, patients should continue forward with new items on the hierarchy until they can remain relaxed when all items from all hierarchies are visualized. When the latter occurs, they will have achieved the feat of having become desensitized to stimuli that formerly provoked fear or anxiety.

There are two ways that systematic desensitization can be used. First, as occurred in the investigation by Miklich and his colleagues (1977), the instructor can present all items from the hierarchies to patients. The role of the patient is to notify the instructor that he or she can either remain relaxed while imagining a stimulus item or that the items continue to elicit fear or anxiety. The instructor can move forward or backward in a hierarchy according to the information provided by a patient. Second, the patient can perform self-directed systematic desensitization. When the patient is relaxed, he or she can imagine the neutral scene. If it can be readily imagined, the patient can proceed to items on a given hierarchy he or she has constructed and written on a 3x5 inch card (usually with the aid of the instructor). The patient can then move forward or backward according to the amount of fear or anxiety that he or she experiences when visualizing a scene.

There are three points that should be noted in using systematic desensitization. First, it is imperative that the patient attain a state of deep muscle relaxation. This is, after all, the behavior that is used to desensitize the patient to the fear-producing stimuli. Second, it is important that the patient visualize both neutral scenes and any of the stimuli presented from the hierarchies. Only the patient knows for certain that he or she can achieve this goal; hence, even if the instructor presents items selected from a hierarchy, the ultimate responsibility for visualizing the stimuli relies upon the patient. Finally, it is important that the patient imagine a scene and still remain relaxed. The patient must not try to please the instructor by saying that an item no longer elicits an emotional response if it still does. By the same token, the instructor must not attempt to move the patient too rapidly through a hierarchy if there are any doubts that the presentation of an item still induces fear or anxiety. If patients perform the procedure by themselves, they should be repeatedly warned not to cheat themselves by moving on through a hierarchy if they still experience an emotional reaction to an item. The procedure of systematic desensitization, in the final analysis, depends entirely upon the patient; he or she can either find it alleviates emotional distress or that the technique does not work for him or her. When the latter occurs, the instructor may wish to go back and repeat part of the procedure to see if success can be attained.

MANAGING ASTHMA ATTACKS

In previous sections, we reviewed a number of strategies the patient might take to help prevent or avoid asthma attacks. Many of these tactics can also be used in managing asthmatic flare-ups. Of particular value would be: (a) establishing self-determined goals; (b) self-assessment; (c) self-reinforcement; (d) making changes in plans to achieve goals; and (e) self-directed stimulus control. In addition, the relaxation strategies and problem solving skills emphasized throughout Asthma Self-Management would be of value in helping manage an asthmatic flare-up.

This discussion will focus on other strategies that may assist patients to manage attacks. These include behavioral and cognitive approaches; accordingly, the discussion is centered around these two major types of techniques.

BEHAVIORAL TECHNIQUES

POSITIVE REINFORCEMENT

This is defined by Martin and Pear (1988) in the following way:

"...if, in a given situation, somebody does something that is followed immediately by a positive reinforcer, then that person is more likely to do the same thing again when he or she next encounters a similar situation" (p. 30).

This is a procedure with which we are all familiar: You know that if you volunteer to do something, such as extra work at the office, and you immediately receive a reinforcer, such as a bonus, you are likely to volunteer for any extra assignment in the future. The patient also knows that if a severe attack is avoided by quickly performing self-management skills, he or she is more likely to perform the same skills the next time the sensations of an asthma flare-up are experienced. We all obey these rules. We all like to receive reinforcers, whether it be something tangible like money, or something that makes us feel good, such as praise for a job well done. The same principle certainly can help patients manage asthma because by helping bring an attack under control, they are reinforced for their action. As noted in the last section, much of the reinforcement received must be provided by the patient. Self-reinforcement is the ability to tell ourselves that we were great in either preventing or managing an attack. **The patient should not be afraid to provide self-reinforcement when he or she performs as taught; it can only increase the probability that he or she will perform in a similar manner in the future with the same positive results.**

Pear and Martin (1988) summarized guidelines for the effective use of positive reinforcement. These include:

1. Selecting the behavior to be reinforced.

   Selecting the behavior to be reinforced is easy: The patient should choose any behavior which helps prevent or manage an asthma attack. If taking maintenance medications helps prevent an attack, then taking the medications should be reinforced. Learning to avoid animals, assuming animal dander triggers attacks, is a behavior that should be selected for reinforcement. Finally, if following a sequence of self-management steps permits the patient to gain control over an attack, he or she should by all means select these behaviors to be reinforced. Each patient is likely to adopt a common set of behaviors, namely self-management skills, in order to prevent or manage an asthma flare-up; at the same time, however, there will be certain behaviors which will help specific individuals to achieve these aims of asthma control. Many of these behaviors will emerge as the patient learns and practices self-management skills; other behaviors may be suggested to the patient by the staff or by personal experiences as he or she participates in Asthma Self-Management.

2. Selecting a reinforcer.

   There are certain rules to follow in selecting a reinforcer. Strong reinforcers are those which are: (a) readily available; (b) can be presented immediately after the desired behavior is performed; (c) can be used repeatedly without producing rapid satiation; and, (d) easy to use. Each patient will select his or her own reinforcers. This the patient can do by writing a list of things that he or she would like to have and is willing to work for by performing the behaviors that have been selected to reinforce. The patient should be certain to always incorporate verbal self-statements along with the use of other types of reinforcement; such self-statements can not only serve as a bridge between behavior and a more tangible reinforcer, but will eventually serve in their own right as the major reinforcer.

3. Applying positive reinforcement.

   Our world is one where much of our behavior is either controlled by punishment, e.g., being audited if we make a mistake on our income tax or fired if we are late to work, or by the avoidance or escape from a potentially punishing situation, e.g., slowing down on the highway if we think we see a police car ahead. Except for the occasional pay check we collect, we do not receive many positive reinforcers for the day-to-day activities we perform, no matter how well we execute them. Positive reinforcement, particularly when applied to personal behavior, can help. It will not only strengthen those behaviors the patient wishes to perform to help control asthma, but it will provide him or her with information as to where he or she is and is going in performing self- management skills. The first time patients notice that the behaviors they performed make a significant contribution to either preventing or managing an attack, they should be thrilled with their efforts. This experience will not only strengthen future performance, but will provide information as to what steps can be performed to contribute to health. Initially, the patient may feel somewhat shy about this action, but, in a world so bereft of positive reinforcement, he or she wants to take advantage of the situation and say, **"Hey, I did a good job!"** This will not only strengthen the behavior performed and make it more likely to be performed in a similar manner under a larger number of conditions, but will also increase the patient's confidence that he or she can, in fact, contribute to the control of asthma.

4. Weaning from the program.

At the beginning, patients may wish to reward themselves with a tangible reinforcer for behaving in a proper manner. Perhaps the purchase of a blouse or a golf club can be contingent upon their performance. Later, however, most of the reinforcement received will come through the positive verbal self-statements a patient makes to himself or herself. **The patient should never hesitate to use positive self-statements as a reinforcer whenever the behavior selected to strengthen has been performed.** Adopting this strategy can be highly effective in insuring future success in performing self-management skills for the control of asthma.

EXTINCTION

This means that when a patient is no longer reinforced for performing a certain behavior, there is the likelihood that there will be a decrease in that behavior. The principle is important to asthmatic patients for two reasons: First, it may be that the patient is performing behaviors that, while once reinforced, no longer contribute to the self-management of asthma. For example, the initial step the patient may take to manage an attack is to telephone the physician and ask for help. If the physician has requested this be done, then the patient should continue the practice; if, however, the physician has requested that self-management steps be taken before placing a call, then the patient's behavior of calling the physician should be extinguished. Be certain that the physician asks that the patient perform self-management skills prior to placing a telephone call before encouraging the patient to extinguish the behavior, however. Second, if reinforcement for performing self-management skills to help manage attacks is not continued, these skills can decrease and eventually be extinguished. Thus, it is important that: (a) self-management skills during asthma attacks are constantly practiced and performed; and (b) performance is reinforced. This will strengthen both the participants' competency and beliefs about their performance. At the same time, these patients' behavior will insure that self-management skills are not extinguished.

Martin and Pear (1988) offer a few suggestions for using extinction:

1. Be specific about the behavior to be extinguished.

It is likely that the patient cannot change all inappropriate behaviors at once. Thus, the patient should select a behavior, such as always telephoning the physician, that should be extinguished first. When the behavior is extinguished, he or she will want to move onto the second behavior to be extinguished, assuming there is one.

2. Monitor the behavior to be extinguished.

This will not only provide the patient with information as to how much the behavior to be extinguished is performed, but with knowledge of what reinforces the behavior. A prime example is the use of emergency rooms by many patients for the treatment of asthma. It is likely that the patient will receive prompt treatment for attacks if they seek the services of an emergency room. For this outcome, the patient is reinforced. However, going to an emergency room for all attacks is not only extremely expensive, but it defeats the purpose of learning to help manage attacks by oneself. If this example is relevant to the patient, the initial consideration would be to monitor how many times he or she goes to a hospital emergency room for the treatment of an attack. When this data is obtained, the acquisition and subsequent performance of self-management skills presents the most likely possibility of changing the event.

3. Implement the plan.

As noted in the above example, if the patient overuses hospital emergency rooms when the physician really doesn't believe the practice necessary, then the patient must extinguish this behavior. We believe that learning to assume more responsibility for attack management, such as that emphasized in Asthma Self-Management, offers the best solution for attaining this goal.

SHAPING

Shaping is a procedure whereby a patient gradually learns, step-by-step, how to perform certain behaviors. The technique is embedded into Asthma Self-Management in that patients are taught, session by session, the steps they should perform to manage their asthma. By proceeding in this manner, new behaviors can be developed by the successive reinforcement of closer approximations to the goal of the self-management of a patient's asthma; at the same time, there should be the extinction of behaviors that interfere with the attainment of this goal.

There are guidelines for using shaping (Martin & Pear, 1988):

1. Select the terminal behavior.

These are selected beforehand for all who go through Asthma Self-Management: Teaching skills required for the self-management of asthma. Reaching these goals involves both the acquisition and subsequent performance of these skills.

2. Select an appropriate reinforcer.

There are several types of reinforcers that are ingrained into Asthma Self-Management. The most salient ones include: (a) the reinforcement received for preventing and managing attacks; (b) the reinforcement received from staff members and physicians for the increased role patients take in attack management;

(c) the reinforcement gained from friends, family members, and classmates for successfully executing self-management skills; and, perhaps most importantly, (d) the self-reinforcement provided through the self-statements made when self-management behaviors have been correctly performed.

3. Implement the plan.

    The plan for shaping behavior is interwoven into Asthma Self-Management. By teaching the patient how to manage asthma a step at a time, self-management skills are gradually learned and the patient has the opportunity to master them through performance.

STIMULUS CONTROL

This technique was described in the last section as the occurrence of a particular behavior in a specific situation. Stimulus control can be important in the management of asthma because there may be distinct environmental stimuli which can help determine whether the patient has been successful in controlling an attack. Three factors of stimulus control which are significant in the management of attacks are:

1. Choose stimuli for determining whether an attack is being alleviated.

    There are two major types of stimuli which can help in deciding whether control over an asthmatic flare-up is being established. First, there are the sensations experienced by a participant. These can be tricky feelings because the patient may sometimes feel better or worse when, in reality, objective indices would show the opposite of what he or she is experiencing. However, by using the peak flow meter, the patient can learn to compare feelings of asthma against the readings obtained from the peak flow meter. Gradually, through the process of shaping, the patient can teach him/herself to correlate sensations of asthma against peak flow readings. The patient will know whether his or her feelings of asthma are correct. Second, peak flow readings obtained with the peak flow meter will tell if obstruction in breathing is still being experienced. If the patient begins blowing higher flow rates, then there is the likelihood that the attack is improving; if, on the other hand, the flow rates continue to drop, the patient will want to institute other self-management procedures to establish control over the episode. Stimulus control here rests upon both feelings and the flow rates obtained with the peak flow meter. When there is agreement between the experiencing of breathing and flow rates, stimulus control has been established which can help control subsequent asthma attacks.

2. Select an appropriate reinforcer.

    There is no need to further elaborate upon the importance of selecting an appropriate reinforcer. As noted in earlier sections, there are a number of ways that behaving in appropriate ways can be reinforced. However, the major method of reinforcement remains self-reinforcement. While not wanting to sound redundant, we can only exclaim that **the patient should always reinforce him/herself after behaving appropriately and there is an improvement in the asthma. The patient helped bring this about; he or she should not be shy about rewarding him/herself for what was done!**

3. Develop discrimination.

In describing the selection of a discriminative stimulus, we pointed out that feelings of an attack do not always coincide with objective measurements of breathing. The patient must develop this discrimination. The way to do so is really fairly simple: First, the patient should judge feelings during an attack and jot down the estimation of what the flow rate would be in using the peak flow meter. Second, he or she should blow into the peak flow meter and compare the flow rate obtained against the number written down beforehand. Finally, if there is little or no disagreement between these two measures, this means there is probably a good correlation between subjective feelings of an attack and the objective peak flow rate. The patient will then want to repeat this procedure during subsequent attacks to be certain this agreement still holds. If, on the other hand, there is a lack of agreement, he or she will want to continually repeat the process until estimates of flow rate are similar to the data obtained with the peak flow meter. In this manner, the patient can learn to accurately estimate the severity of an attack. This knowledge, in turn, will permit more effectiveness in using self-management procedures to control asthma.

CHAINING

With this procedure, a series of behaviors or steps is linked together to achieve an aim. Central to Asthma Self-Management is teaching management of attacks in a stepwise fashion; for this reason, the patient should already have a solid notion of chaining.

There are certain ways that the ability to use chaining in performing self-management procedures can be enhanced. These would include:

1. Step-by-step performance of self-management procedures.

The patient has been taught to try one step to see if it helps alleviate asthma. If the initial step does not work, the patient has been instructed to initiate the second step and so on until the attack is controlled. For many attacks, the patient will want to stick to this stepwise procedure to bring an asthmatic flare-up under control; at other times, especially during severe attacks, he or she may want to leap ahead to contact the physician or, in extreme cases, to go immediately to the hospital. The patient should remain flexible in deciding the best course of action to take.

2. Reinforce the stepwise strategy for managing attacks.

We cannot emphasize enough the need to reinforce the patient for taking the proper steps to help bring an attack under control. In many cases, reinforcement will be provided by others, including the physician, medical personnel, friends, family members, etc. In other cases, however, the patient must use self-reinforcement to strengthen the ability to proceed step-by-step through the procedure in order to bring the attack under control. When this occurs, we cannot emphasize too much that **the patient reinforce himself/herself! The patient has done something to help control asthma and deserves such a reward!**

GENERALIZATION

There are two kinds of generalization: Stimulus generalization and response generalization. Stimulus generalization means that behaviors, such as those involved in managing an attack, become more likely in a second situation if they have been reinforced in another situation. In other words, if the patient is successful at using self-management procedures to help control an attack at home and is reinforced for doing so, it is likely that the same procedures will be effective if used by the patient at work. Response generalization means that a behavior becomes more probable in a situation as a result of it being strengthened in the presence of that situation. In other words, when the patient is successful at performing self-management skills at home, these behaviors will be strengthened when he or she uses them to help manage other attacks that occur in the same environment. Thus, in stimulus generalization, there is an increased likelihood of using self-management procedures across settings if they prove successful at helping control an attack in one setting and reinforcement is received, including self-reinforcement, for the behavior; in response generalization, there is an increased likelihood that self-management skills will be performed more in the future when they prove successful in assisting the patient to control an asthmatic episode and he or she is reinforced for the behavior.

There are two ways to improve generalization of behavior. First, it is important that the performance of self-management skills is constantly practiced. The more they are practiced, the more proficient the patient will become at performing these skills. The more proficient the patient is, the more reinforcement he or she should receive. This will mean that the responses entailed in self-management will become stronger and stronger; the patient will find that he or she does make a significant contribution to the overall management of asthma. Second, the patient should not hesitate to try out newly-developed self-management skills in other settings and situations. When the patient finds they work well at home, he or she should try them somewhere like a shopping center. The stronger the skills and the more settings they are applied to, the more valuable they are to the patient. **The patient should practice self-management skills at every opportunity. He or she should always remember to reinforce when the efforts assist in the management of the episode!**

AVOIDANCE AND ESCAPE

Avoidance means that every effort is made to avoid the occurrence of an aversive stimulus. In the case of asthma, it means that the patient avoids, whenever possible, the occurrence of a trigger of asthma. Escape means that the removal of certain stimuli, such as punishers, following the occurrence of a response will strengthen and increase the likelihood that the removal or escape response will occur in the future. With asthma, this simply means that when a response to escape from a precipitant of asthma is made, the escape performance will be strengthened.

Avoidance and escape are very important in the overall management of asthma. If the patient knows the triggers of asthma and is able to either avoid them or, when they occur, to escape from them, this is half of the battle. He or she may be able to prevent an attack from occurring or, in the event one does occur, be able to keep it from intensifying in severity.

COGNITIVE TECHNIQUES

ELLIS'S RATIONAL-EMOTIVE RESTRUCTURING

This approach, derived from the work of Albert Ellis (1973), is based on the premise that there is a close connection between what we say to ourselves and how we feel. Most daily emotional problems and behaviors, he believes, stem from irrational statements we make to ourselves when events in our lives are not quite the way we would like them to be. We tend to grasp on to irrational beliefs which consistently generate emotional disturbance for us. Common illogical ideas have been noted by Ellis (1973). They include:

1. The idea that it is a necessity for all of us to be loved or approved by virtually every significant person in our lives.

2. The idea that we should always be thoroughly competent, adequate, and achieve in all possible respects in order for us to consider ourselves worthwhile.

3. The idea that certain people are bad, wicked, or villainous, and that they should be severely blamed and punished for their evil.

4. The idea that it is awful and catastrophic when things are not the way one would like them to be (Ellis is particularly concerned about our ability to "catastrophize," and to tell ourselves that events are so bad that we can't possibly cope with them).

5. The idea that our unhappiness is caused by external factors out of our control, and that we have little or no ability to control our terrors and disturbances.

6. The idea that it is easier to avoid than to face our difficulties and responsibilities.

7. The idea that our past history is an all-important determinant of our present behavior and that, because something once affected our life, it will definitely continue to do so.

Ellis believes there are ways to overcome these thoughts which seem to control so much of our lives. Suggestions include:

1. Review each idea with respect to how it influences us.

2. Monitor ourselves and record any self-defeating thoughts or ideas. They often occur involuntarily and at key moments; hence, we must be vigilant in self-monitoring our feelings and thoughts. Self-defeating thoughts can certainly undermine our performance of self-management skills to control asthma.

3. Record these thoughts on a regular basis, much as the patient records data on the asthma diary each day.

4. Identify stressful events and note any negative thoughts associated with them. We may find that certain thoughts and feelings frequently occur at times when we are upset.

5. Try to counteract irrational and negative thoughts with positive and realistic statements.

Another approach suggested by Ellis is the A-B-C method. Basically, this asks that we think of negative thoughts according to the following paradigm:

A = The Activating Experience. This usually involves some sort of personal disappointment. An example would be that we feel depressed because our asthma was not brought under control as effectively as we wished. However, according to Ellis, this could not be true because failure to control an episode could not cause an emotional consequence (Rudestam, 1980).

B = The Belief System. This shapes the consequence more directly. The Belief System has both a rational and irrational component:

a. **The rational component** is empirically valid and is a positive coping response; it can lead to feelings of disappointment and sorrow as a result of the Activating Experience, but not to intense feelings of worthlessness, guilt, or depression. The rational component is empirically valid and is a positive coping response (Rudestam, 1980).

b. **The irrational component** creates worthless evaluations and hopelessness about the future. This belief is unrealistic since it suggests we should never experience any type of loss or disappointment.

C = Emotional Consequences. These are the feelings we experience such as depression, guilt, or sorrow. The tendency of most people is to credit these feelings to A, the Activating Experience. However, this is an incorrect assumption in that the Activating Experience cannot ever directly cause an Emotional Consequence in another individual, including ourselves.

There are various ways of managing the A-B-C paradigm. One method is to categorize events into the following system: (a) the situation; (b) the feelings experienced; (c) the thoughts about the matter; and (d) alternative interpretations. In thinking through possible alternative situations, we can begin to see where we have catastrophized or overreacted to the situation. We can also see how self-management skills might help us better control such situations in the future.

BECK'S COGNITIVE THERAPY

Beck has independently developed a system similar to that of Ellis. He thinks that many of us engage excessively in aberrant, fallacious, or dysfunctional thinking; this behavior, in turn, contributes to our problems. Among the various types of dysfunctional thinking Beck identifies are:

1. **Dichotomous thinking.** This is the tendency to think in absolute terms. For example, if the patient finds self-management skills do not help control a given attack, he or she may think, "These techniques are not for me. They don't work." This may be totally incorrect; the attack may have intensified more had the patient not performed self-management skills.

2. **Arbitrary inference.** This is drawing a conclusion on the basis of inadequate evidence. Referring to the last example, the patient might say, "I did not perform self-management skills right." In reality, as we noted, the attack would have been more severe had he or she not taken the action.

3. **Overgeneralization.** This is reaching a general conclusion on the basis of too few examples. We all overgeneralize from time to time. The patient might think that every time he or she is exposed to a precipitant of asthma, such as exercise, an attack will be experienced. However, this is an overgeneralization: It may not be exercise per se that triggers an episode, but the degree to which one exercises.

4. **Magnification.** This is the process of exaggerating the meaning or significance of a particular event. A common example is that presented by panic and asthma. Many people are frightened during attacks and, in some cases, they panic. However, just because the patient panics once does not mean that he or she will experience the same degree of fear or anxiety in the future. Much of what occurs in the future will depend upon practice and performance of self-management skills. As the patient becomes proficient at these skills, the likelihood that panic will be experienced during these attacks will decrease.

The ways Beck suggests we manage dysfunctional thinking are:

a. To identify clearly the dysfunctional thoughts and maladaptive assumptions that are causing our problem.

b. To test these thoughts against reality by hypothesis testing. This will reveal the extent to which such thoughts are dysfunctional.

c. To make every effort to change the dysfunctional thinking through reality testing.

d. To be certain to provide reinforcement to ourselves when we do change our cognitions so that they are more in line with reality.

MEICHENBAUM'S SELF-INSTRUCTIONAL METHODS

We have discussed self-instructional methods to a great degree in this chapter. Meichenbaum (1986) asks that when we recognize our negative self-statements, we use more realistic, positive statements. In addition, Meichenbaum advocates the use of the relaxation exercises that have been taught to cope with negative and self-defeating thoughts and feelings. Meichenbaum also uses what he calls "stress inoculations." In self-management, this might take the form of the patient imaging stressful scenes surrounding asthma and attempting to relax while imaging such scenes (much as the patient may have done if he or she applied systematic desensitization). This practice can help later to cope with stress. As usual, practice in stress inoculation can strengthen the ability to manage attacks; in addition, the patient always wants to **reinforce when he or she has successfully coped with a situation that formerly elicited stress.**

THOUGHT STOPPING

There are times when it is difficult to stop thinking about some thought or feeling. Wolpe (1958) suggested a technique called "thought stopping" which may be of benefit. This involves three steps:

1. Think about the problem thought or feeling.

2. When you have a clear image of this problem, yell "STOP" to yourself. This serves as punishment for your cognitive behavior.

3. Eventually fade out the use of the word, "STOP," when you find you no longer ruminate about the problem thought or feeling. As usual, **reinforce yourself for your achievement!**

THOUGHT CONTROL

A number of psychologists (e.g., Meichenbaum, 1986; Suinn, 1986) have discussed using thought control. Suinn (1986) has described the separate use of both negative and positive thoughts. Both approaches can help with the management of asthma.

Negative Thoughts

Suinn (1986) suggests the following ways to use negative thoughts:

1. In many instances, negative thoughts seem to have a life of their own; they consume much of our conscious thought and interfere with our lives. Instead of letting these thoughts feed on themselves, try and use them to work out a solution. Suinn (1986) suggests we try and turn a negative thought into a positive event not by ignoring the thought, but by trying to use it to induce positive and corrective behavior.

2. There are ways of coping with intruding and negative thoughts. We might consider the following approaches.

   a. Examine them to see if they can be used in a positive way to work out a solution. The patient may experience a thought or feeling (such as a nagging fear that he or she will not use self-management skills correctly during an upcoming flare-up) that can be changed by practicing these skills more before an attack. This is a positive use of negative thoughts: They spur us to improve our overall performance.

   b. Analyze the source of the thoughts and take action to remove their origins. We all monitor ourselves very well. In the case of negative thoughts, we will want to carefully analyze our thoughts to determine whether we can pinpoint the antecedent factors leading to these responses. As was noted earlier, it is important that we be realistic and sensible in making such decisions. It could be that there is no realistic basis for the thoughts. The patient has repeatedly shown that he or she can perform self-management skills and they help control asthma. When doubts occur, the patient again should practice the skills more; as usual, **the patient should reinforce when the skills are performed correctly.**

c. Try and replace negative thoughts with plans for adapting to the future. The patient may wish to change goals or to set new ones to work towards. Then, begin working to achieve these goals.

d. Consider alternative points of view. The patient is beginning to demonstrate that he or she can make a significant contribution to the management of asthma. He or she should remember back to when self-management skills were not known and his/her asthma was totally under the control of others. We can all be hard on ourselves from time to time. However, the patient need not be if he or she is performing self-management skills to help control asthma. The patient is beginning to emerge as a major ingredient in the control of the disorder.

e. Review strengths and how they are to be applied. The patient should always consider the strengths he or she has developed in the period he or she has been involved with Asthma Self-Management. These thoughts will reinforce the patient and help erase any self-doubts he or she may have about his/her performance in the future. Continuing to expand upon or to refine self-management skills can also help in coping with negative thoughts.

f. A neutral thought can often be substituted for the bothersome, interfering thought. Earlier, we asked that the patient think of neutral scenes, such as a pleasant stroll through the autumn countryside or viewing a favorite television program, as neutral scenes to use when anxious and unable to relax. The patient should imagine these same scenes when bothered by a troublesome thought; this can help both to relax and to consider thoughts within a more realistic perspective.

g. Contain negative thoughts that seem resistant to change. Suinn (1986) suggests we consider one of two strategies: First, the exercises described earlier for thought stopping can be used; this can help block thoughts from further intruding into the consciousness. Second, let the thoughts move freely in and out of the mind until they can be isolated away from the consciousness. When the patient has succeeded with either approach, he or she should not forget to **reinforce.**

Positive Thoughts

We have emphasized the acquisition of positive thoughts throughout Asthma Self-Management. Without such thoughts, it is unlikely that the patient will make a sustained effort to change behavior. The strategies suggested by Suinn (1986) for creating positive thoughts are very similar to those suggested by others for creating sound psychological attitudes. They include:

1. The patient should value him/herself as a person who happens to have asthma. No one is perfect; everyone has some sort of problem they have to consider whether it be poor eyesight or an inability to obtain a job. Always try to make the best of the situation. It doesn't hurt to note one more time that successful practice of self-management skills can do nothing but enhance the perceptions one has of himself or herself as a valuable and worthwhile person.

2. The patient should know where he or she is with self-management skills before experiencing asthma. It is always important to be able to know beforehand exactly what skills the patient believes he or she can perform both before and during an attack. The patient does not want to sell him/herself short by thinking that he or she cannot perform certain skills when it has successfully been done in the past. On the other hand, the patient does not want to overestimate his or her ability to control what may be a severe asthma flare-up. With experience at performing self-management skills, the patient will have a good idea of the level of experience. It is important that he or she continually evaluate the level of experience, and be realistic in making such an evaluation. Often, the patient will have the tendency to downplay experience in that he or she is far more capable of managing attacks than he or she gives himself/herself credit for. At other times, however, the patient may think he or she can do more than is called for in order for the attack to be controlled. The determination of the level of skills is one that the patient will need to make for himself or herself. The methods we have taught in decision-making and problem-solving should assist in this task.

3. The patient should review the programs from where he or she started to where he or she has progressed. The patient should try to always keep progress in perspective. The patient knows that he or she is more skilled and confident than before participating in Asthma Self-Management. Each successful performance of skills in helping control an attack should further enhance the patient's confidence. At the same time, there may be an occasional setback--the attack that from the outset requires more intensive care than the patient can provide--which should not deter in any way from the overall performance by the patient. These are but slight impediments, like the daily bumps in our lives, which can be overcome by successfully executing self-management skills to manage the next asthma flare-up that is experienced.

4. The patient should know what he or she wants, what his or her goals are, and the reasons for wanting to do well. It is doubtful that the patient would have entered into Asthma Self-Management had he or she not had certain expectations and goals for participation. As the patient learns and performs self-management skills, goals continue to evolve. The patient will come to believe that much of the effort for controlling an attack does not rest with external factors, such as a hospital emergency room, but with himself or herself. This realization cannot help but elicit positive thoughts about the ability to help manage asthma.

IMAGERY

There are a number of ways to use imagery in the self-management of asthma. One major use of imagery is to help the patient visualize more clearly the problem or problems he or she wants to solve. By managing a problem beforehand, the patient can plan and rehearse ways to cope with an attack when it actually occurs. There are two general approaches to imagery which will be presented here: The first represents a general approach used by many different therapists; the second represents a more detailed approach suggested by Suinn (1976;1986).

General Imagery Instructions

The successful use of imagery involves a number of steps, several of which the patient already knows. The major ingredients of imagery would involve the following steps:

1. The patient should practice the deep muscle relaxation exercises he or she has already been taught. The patient wants to be able to relax on self-cue when he or she wishes to do so.

2. After the patient has achieved a level of relaxation, he or she should make a suggestion to himself or herself. This should be direct and positive such as the following, "I know I can help control my asthma." Repetition is important in making this post-relaxation suggestion; make the suggestion several times. If mental imagery can be formed and added to the verbal suggestion, it will make the suggestion more potent. Thus, after the patient is relaxed and has made suggestions to himself or herself, he or she forms a mental picture of himself or herself performing a self-management skill with vigor and confidence.

3. The patient does not want to overload himself or herself with too many suggestions at once; rather, it is better only to repeat the same suggestion several times.

4. Suggestions should be worded with the goal the patient has set for himself or herself in mind. Always be certain that suggestions incorporate the desired result of the action.

5. Mental imagery training involves that the patient imagine himself or herself performing self-management skills perfectly before actually attempting such performance. When the patient has performed self-management skills well, engaging in mental imagery to reconstruct what was done can be valuable. It also permits the patient to make self-statements to **reinforce himself or herself.**

6. The patient should exercise mental practice and imagery training. The best results with imagery are obtained when the patient can view himself or herself from the inside with eyes open or closed. This permits the patient to see and feel the way through an activity as he or she can actually visualize what it is he or she is doing. This approach will also assist in later spotting and feeling reactions during the actual performance of self-management skills.

7. There are other important factors which are helpful in improving ability to use imagery. Those that seem significant in helping in the performance of self-management skills to an optimal level include:

   a. The patient should mentally rehearse self-management skills in the environment where he or she thinks such skills to manage asthma will later be performed. If most of the attacks occur at home, the patient should mentally rehearse self-management skills while at home; later, he or she will want to generalize the performance by mentally rehearsing these skills in other settings.

   b. Any mentally-rehearsed activity should be practiced in its entirety. In using self-management skills, the patient wants to proceed, one step at a time, from the time the attack is detected until it has been aborted. He or she should mentally rehearse the performance of these skills in the same manner.

c.   The mental practice performed must be successful. The patient wants to be certain that, in imagining the performance of self-management skills, he or she achieves the aim of helping control an asthmatic episode.

d.   At least one mental practice should precede the actual performance of the activity the patient wishes to perform. With self-management of an asthma attack, it is important that the patient practice the performance of these skills in the imagination before an attack occurs and he or she must perform these skills.

e.   The mental practice of an activity should be performed at the same speed with which the patient would perform the skills in the real-life setting. This is important: If the patient is performing the steps required to control an attack, he or she can learn the rhythm of what to do by being certain to imagine that he or she is performing a step, permitting time to see if the step alleviates the flare-up, performing the second step, etc.

f.   In performing mental practice, the patient should concentrate on imagining the "feel" of the action. The patient wants to know how it feels to perform one step and its likely consequences, the feel of the second step, etc.

8. Psychological coping skills can be developed in that mental imagery permits the imagination of scenes or situations which are not likely to be replicated in a real-life setting. The patient can be free-wheeling and imagining himself or herself performing self-management skills under all types of situations and circumstances. The patient may never actually experience an attack under some conditions, say at the top of Mount Everest, but at least he or she can imagine what to do under these circumstances. In addition, there are two other types of coping skills that can be developed through imagery:

a.   The patient can correct any errors that he or she thinks are likely to occur when an asthma attack is later experienced. Imagining the performance permits the patient to detect what skills may require change before he or she actually experiences an attack.

b.   Through mental imagery, the patient can not only set goals for himself or herself, but can refine the goals already established. A goal is whatever the patient makes it; mental imagery can help the patient establish what he or she thinks would be realistic goals to aim for in real life.

VISUAL-MOTOR BEHAVIOR REHEARSAL

This program, originally developed to improve the performance of athletes (Suinn, 1976; 1986), has components which are appropriate to the self-management of any type of problem, including asthma. The patient already knows, in fact, most of these skills. It is recombining them in a different way that is required for visual-motor behavior rehearsal (VMBR). Seven stages of VMBR include:

1. There are two major aspects in the first stage of VMBR; the patient must know them both. First, the patient is asked to relax on self-cue. Through deep muscle relaxation training, he or she already can achieve this goal. Second, the patient is asked to imagine a pleasant scene, such as a walk outdoors or watching television. The purpose of Stage I is that the patient alternates these activities at will; this helps stamp in ability to control body and thoughts.

2. This stage is similar to the first in that the patient alternately practices relaxation and imagery. In addition, however, the patient now adds the imagery of successfully performing self-management skills. The patient wants to imagine him/herself performing at this level as thoroughly as possible (he or she also wants to **reinforce** for such images).

3. There is also little difference between Step 3 and the previous two steps. Here, the patient imagines him/herself as he or she successfully performed self-management skills to help control past attacks. The patient wants to imagine this scene several times, but intersperse it with thoughts of a pleasant scene or being relaxed. The purpose of the scene is to teach the patient to switch back and forth from relaxing the body to imagining a pleasant scene to visualizing how self-management skills to control asthma have been used successfully. The ability to move from activity to activity can enhance the performance in later managing attacks.

4. This step is identical to that followed in deep muscle relaxation. Basically, the patient wants to imagine that he or she is experiencing asthma while attempting to relax. When the patient has successfully relaxed, he or she again wants to visualize experiencing an asthmatic flare-up. By alternating these activities, the patient can again sharpen the ability to relax, imagine scenes, and visually work through an attack according to the self-instructions he or she provides him/herself.

5. This step is similar to what was described earlier: The patient wants to select a situation where an attack is likely to be experienced and visualize him/herself using self-management skills to help bring it under control. The patient should be certain to command him/herself to take whatever action is required; this will sharpen the ability to later deal with an asthmatic flare-up.

6. The patient has selected goals he or she wishes to attain to help control asthma. These goals may be accompanied by key phrases or attitudes such as, "I can do it," or "I did it well in the past." In this step of VMBR, these phrases are added to the visualization of using self-management procedures to help control asthma. These positive thoughts can not only help motivate the patient to perform well, but they provide a certain degree of reinforcement. Thus, the patient wants to use such positive phrases or attitudes during attacks.

7. The final step suggests visual practice of self-management skills over and over so that, during future attacks, the patient has a strong edge over the disorder. The patient will know what he or she expects to do and, more than likely, will act in accordance with his or her expectations. Knowing and performing self-management skills provides the patient with a major edge over asthma; it will be up to the patient to further increase this edge as the performance of these skills is perfected.

References

Beck, A. T., Rush, A. J., Shaw, B. F., & Emery, G. (1967). Cognitive therapy of depression. New York: Guilford.

Benson, H. (1975). The relaxation response. New York: Morrow.

Ellis, A. (1973). Humanistic psychotherapy. New York: McGraw-Hill.

Martin, G., & Pear, J. (1988). Behavior modification: What it is and how to do it. Englewood Cliffs, NJ: Prentice-Hall.

Meichenbaum, D. (1986). Cognitive behavior modification. In F. H. Kanfer & A. P. Goldstein (Eds.), Helping people change: A textbook of methods, 3rd edition, 346-380. New York: Pergamon.

Miklich, D. R., Renne, C. M., Creer, T. L., Alexander, A. B., Chai, H., Davis, M. H., Hoffman, A., & Danker-Brown, P. (1977). The clinical utility of behavior therapy as an adjunctive treatment for asthma. Journal of Allergy & Clinical Immunology, 60, 285-294.

Rudestam, K. E. (1980). Methods of self-change: An ABC primer. Monterey, CA: Brooks/Cole Publishing Company.

Schultz, J. H., & Luthe, W. (1959). Autogenic training. New York: Grune & Stratton.

Suinn, R. M. (1976). Visual-motor behavior rehearsal for adaptive behavior. In J. Krumboltz & C. Thoresen (Eds.), Counseling methods. New York: Holt, Rinehart & Winston.

Suinn, R. M. (1986). Seven steps to peak performance. Lewiston, NY: Hans Huber Publishers.

Wolpe, J. (1958). Psychotherapy by reciprocal inhibition. Stanford, CA: Stanford University Press.

SIGNS OF WORSENING ASTHMA
Visual 4.1

Voice Changes

Swollen Face

Shallow and/or Fast Breathing

Quickening Pulse

Listless Behavior/Extreme Fatigue

Difficult Breathing/Shortness of Breath

Audible Wheezing/Whistling While Breathing

SIGNS OF SEVERE ASTHMA
Visual 4.2

Breathing from the neck up

Raised shoulders

Indentation at the hollow of the neck

Sweating

Flared nostrils

Hands over head

Blue lips and/or fingernails

Labored breathing

ASTHMA SELF-MANAGEMENT STEPS

Visual 4.3

1. REST AND RELAXATION

    A. Deep Breathing

    B. Deep Muscle Relaxation

2. DRINK WARM LIQUIDS

3. USE MEDICATIONS PRESCRIBED FOR
    ATTACKS

4. CONTACT FAMILY OR FRIENDS IF AN
    ATTACK DOES NOT ABATE

5. CALL YOUR PHYSICIAN OR SEEK
    EMERGENCY MEDICAL HELP

Step 1a

REST AND RELAXATION:

Visual 4.4

1. Lie on the floor or bed

    Bend knees

    Keep feet flat on floor

    Put one hand on chest, other hand on

    stomach

2. Close eyes, and turn attention towards

    breathing

3. Breathe in through nose while pushing

    stomach out

4. Blow air out through mouth and

    pursed lips

5. Use the hand on your stomach to help

    you push the air out

Step 1b
<u>Deep Muscle Relaxation</u>
Visual 4.5

Tense and relax muscles in the following sequence:

Hands, lower arms

Upper arms, shoulders

Scalp, forehead, eyes

Eyes, nose, mid-facial muscles

Lower facial muscles, jaw, mouth

Neck

Chest, shoulders, upper back

Lower back, stomach

Buttocks, hips

Thighs

Lower leg, calf

Feet

Review all muscles in your mind's eye

Step 2

DRINK WARM LIQUIDS
Visual 4.6

1. Warm liquids help relax and open up the airways.

2. Warm liquids help thin the mucus and replace lost water.

Step 3

<u>USE MEDICATIONS PRESCRIBED</u>

<u>FOR ATTACKS</u>
Visual 4.7

If relaxation and drinking warm liquids have not

prevented or controlled an attack, take the

medications prescribed for an attack by

your physician.

Be sure that you understand which medications

are specifically for use during an attack and

which medications are for daily use to

prevent attacks

Some medications, used to <u>prevent</u> attacks,

will make the attack worse if taken <u>during</u>

an attack.

Step 4

<u>CONTACT FAMILY OR FRIENDS</u>
Visual 4.8

EDUCATE FAMILY AND FRIENDS ABOUT THE FIVE ASTHMA SELF-MANAGEMENT STEPS

CALL FAMILY OR FRIENDS WHEN YOU NEED HELP WITH INITIATING ATTACK MANAGEMENT STEPS OR GETTING EMERGENCY MEDICAL SERVICES

EDUCATE FAMILY MEMBERS OR FRIENDS AS TO WHEN TO CONTACT EMERGENCY HELP FOR YOU; THEY SHOULD KNOW THE SIGNS OF SEVERE ASTHMA

Step 5

CONTACT A PHYSICIAN/

SEEK EMERGENCY MEDICAL HELP

Visual 4.9

Signs of severe asthma, such as blue lips or fingernails, shallow breathing, or having your sole attention focused on breathing, indicate you should seek immediate medical help.

Breathing is Life: If in doubt, CALL A PHYSICIAN.

SESSION FIVE
CONSEQUENCES OF ASTHMA

GOALS
1. To discuss problems that arise as the result of having asthma.
2. To introduce problem-solving strategies for coping with the consequences of asthma.

EQUIPMENT
Name tags.
Paper and pencils for all participants.
Overhead projector.

SUPPLIES
Coffee, tea, snacks, or light lunch.

SESSION FIVE OUTLINE

TOPIC/ ACTIVITY	REQUIRED MATERIAL	APPROXIMATE TIME ALLOWED
Welcome & salutations	Name tags	5 Minutes
Questions about prior sessions/ readings		10 Minutes
Adding imagery to the relaxation exercise	Reclining chairs or bedrolls and pillows	20 Minutes
Psychological responses to asthma	Visual 5.1, 5.2	
Family responses to asthma	Visual 5.3	
Lifestyle changes	Visual 5.4	
Physical changes	Visual 5.5	
Economic costs	Visual 5.6	
Homework	Practice relaxation twice daily; SOLVED Problems exercise, Visual 5.7, read Chapter 7	10 Minutes

SESSION FIVE TEACHING NOTES

Welcome and Salutations

Provide a name tag to each participant. Allow time for small talk by group members prior to getting into the session material.

Questions About Prior Sessions/Readings

Allow time to ask questions about material covered earlier in the program.

Relaxation Exercise with Imagery

Give everyone a chance to share their experience with practicing the relaxation exercise. Review the basics of preparation, deep breathing, and deep muscle relaxation. Discuss the rationale for including imagery in relaxation exercises. Conduct the relaxation exercise contained in Chapter 6 of the participant manual. Be sure to allow group members to express all misgivings or concerns about practicing relaxation. The leader and group members may help individuals develop alternative approaches to relaxation (e.g., meditation, yoga).

Consequences of Asthma

There are no easy solutions for most of the problem consequences of asthma. The suggestions listed are provided as guidelines to generate group discussion. The best guide for discussing these items is by developing a thorough understanding of the concepts that have been presented in earlier sessions. Although most concerns can be solved by you and the group members, if someone reveals a situation that you feel unqualified to discuss, suggest a professional counselor or therapist be consulted.

The consequences of asthma have been divided into five major categories: psychological responses, responses of family and friends, lifestyle changes, physical changes, and economic costs. Allow the group to generate as many consequences and solutions as possible before filling in missing information. Welcome their suggestions and stimulate discussion to elicit innovative ways to deal with these problems (See Visuals 5.1-5.6). Often the discussion of the consequences of asthma will extend into sessions six and seven. Visual 5.2, on the fear of dying of asthma, can stimulate considerable discussion; this fear is a common concern that most asthmatic patients rarely take the opportunity to talk about.

Homework

There are two parts to this week's homework. *First*, group members should continue to practice relaxation at least once (preferably twice) per day. Instruct them to use the relaxation exercise which includes the use of imagery when they feel they have mastered the deep breathing/ relaxation exercise. *Second,* participants should choose one consequence of asthma which they would like to change. Instruct them to devise a strategy to prevent or lessen the impact of that consequence. If time permits, have them select which consequence they wish to work on prior to the end of this session. Remind them that they will be asked to share with the group their experiences in trying to make the desired change. Provide as much encouragement as possible. Remind participants that Chapters 7 and 8 should be read before the next session.

SESSION FIVE BACKGROUND READING

MANAGING CONSEQUENCES OF ASTHMA

In some ways, these are the most difficult problems to manage because they are often insidious: One may not realize that they exist. These problems can take the form of co-workers who think the patient suffers from a contagious disease to a relative who thinks the patient's respiratory distress is all in the head. We have described the various types of consequences apt to be experienced as a result of asthma. Ways to manage these consequences have been suggested in the client manual. There are other problems, however, that will occur from time to time and be unique to the patient. While there are no sure-fire ways to alter these consequences, a few suggestions can be offered. These provide techniques for not only preventing, managing, or altering the courses of asthma, but serve to review some of the basic principles we have already described in the program. These principles, most of which were summarized by Watson and Tharp (1989), are (Table 5:1):

TABLE 5:1. MANAGING THE CONSEQUENCES OF ASTHMA (INCLUDING SUGGESTIONS BY WATSON & THARP, 1989)

Self-statements act as powerful guides to behavior.

Operant behavior is a function of its consequences.

A positive reinforcer maintains and strengthens behavior.

A negative reinforcer strengthens behavior by its removal.

Punished behavior will occur less often.

Behaviors no longer reinforced will extinguish.

Intermittent reinforcement increases resistance to extinction.

Most operant behavior is guided by antecedent stimuli.

An antecedent can be a signal for an unpleasant event.

Through conditioning, antecedents can elicit automatic responses that are often emotional.

Many behaviors are learned by observing others.

Patients should always use self-reinforcement when they successfully perform self-management skills.

Principle I: From early life to adulthood, self-statements act as powerful guides to behavior.

This point has been emphasized throughout Asthma Self-Management. While professionals initially determine the type of treatment the patient receives for asthma, the patient has gradually taken over more responsibility for the management of many of his or her attacks. Behaviors that are affected by their consequences are referred to as operant behaviors. This means that the skills performed operate on asthma to produce better control of the disorder. In the future, the patient is more likely to use self-statements to direct and guide him or her in the performance of skills required to control asthma. In this respect, there will be an increase in the behaviors performed that directly operate upon asthma.

Principle II: Operant behavior is a function of its consequences.

No matter what you do, your behaviors will be strengthened or weakened by events that follow them. If the patient performs behaviors that help manage asthma, it is probable that he or she will be more likely to perform these behaviors in the future. A consequence that strengthens a behavior is referred to as a positive reinforcer. We have repeatedly urged patients to reinforce themselves when an act has been performed that contributes to the successful management of asthma; the response can do nothing but strengthen their performance during future attacks.

Principle III: A positive reinforcer is a consequence that maintains and strengthens behavior by its presence.

A positive reinforcer is anything that strengthens the preceding behavior. Positive reinforcers may be anything; the list is exhaustive and very personalized. Praise from both others and patients for successfully performing self-management skills acts as a reinforcing consequence; it can also serve as an antecedent event in helping the patient to initiate future self-management strategies.

Principle IV: A negative reinforcer is an unpleasant consequence that strengthens behavior by being removed from the situation.

There are few consequences that are more unpleasant than being unable to breathe. The patient has learned to escape or avoid unpleasant consequences through personal performance. **Escape learning**, as we noted, refers to the behaviors or skills that terminate an unpleasant situation. Each time skills are performed that help bring an asthma attack under control, an unpleasant consequence, namely an asthma flare-up, is escaped. There may be few more effective consequences, even though they are unpleasant, that can help control behavior. **Avoidance learning**, as also noted, refers to behaviors that prevent the possibility of an unpleasant consequence. If potential triggers of attacks can be avoided, avoidance learning has been successfully practiced. Clearly, we have stressed, the patient's behavior is affected by the reinforcement he or she receives. Patients are reinforced for what they do. If patients do something that helps control asthma, they should receive positive reinforcement. When patients avoid or escape from unpleasant situations, they deserve reinforcement. We have often found that patients with asthma were more proud of their ability to prevent attacks than they were of aborting asthmatic flare-ups.

Principle V: Behavior that is punished will occur less often.

While going through Asthma Self-Management, patients will come to realize that they can punish themselves by needlessly exposing themselves to known precipitants of asthma and inducing an attack. A patient may find that if exercise is not monitored carefully, for example, he or she could end up with asthma. This may produce a decrease in exercise habits, although we hope that it doesn't. What we hope the patient learns is that the lack of self-monitoring of the amount of exercise engaged in was the problem. Under these circumstances, the patient should show a decrease in the number of times he or she failed to monitor exercise carefully. Punishment can also occur when behavior leads to the loss of something pleasant. An example is that patients may be looking forward to a pleasant outing with their families when they knowingly expose themselves to a precipitant--dusting the house for a family reunion seems a likely bet--that leads to asthma. Under these circumstances, we hope that the attack does not lead a patient to want to decrease future family reunions; we do hope, however, that it leads to a decrease in the tendency the patient may have to personally do all of the housework even though it can lead to respiratory distress.

Principle VI: Behaviors no longer reinforced will fade.

This is a principle that we must stress: The patient will undoubtedly find that self-management skills can provide considerable value to help gain control over asthmatic episodes. When this occurs, the patient will be reinforced for the responses. However, if the patient fails to practice these skills, they eventually will not be reinforced and the patient will find that he or she no longer makes a contribution to asthma management. Under these circumstances, it could be said that the behavior has been extinguished. To prevent this from occurring, it is imperative that self-management skills continue to be practiced and performed long after participation in this program is terminated. This practice will not only sharpen skills, thus permitting the patient to make a greater contribution to the management of asthma, but he or she will continue to be reinforced by the success of the performance. There is little likelihood that there will be a decrement in the performance of self-management skills under these circumstances; there will be even less of a chance of extinction of self-management skills occurring.

Principle VII: Intermittent reinforcement increases resistance to extinction.

At first, we ask patients to reinforce themselves each time an attack has been successfully managed through the performance of self-management skills. After awhile, when a patient is both competent and confident about the use of these skills, he or she may need only occasional reinforcement. The patient knows that behavior helps control asthma, and expects that it will continue to do so in the future. Under such circumstances, intermittent reinforcement is all that is necessary to maintain performance.

Principle VIII: Most operant behavior is eventually guided by antecedent stimuli or cues.

In this situation, patients are aware that antecedent conditions can trigger attacks. The flare-ups, in turn, warrant that self-management procedures be applied to bring the episode under control. If attacks can be prevented by avoiding known stimuli, a patient is much better off than if he or she has to treat an incipient attack. When the latter occurs, however, the patient is more likely to establish control over the episode if he or she escapes from the trigger of the episode and initiates self-management procedures.

Principle IX: An antecedent can be a cue or signal that an unpleasant event may be imminent.

There are a number of signals which may warn the patient that an asthma attack may be experienced. Common signals include: (a) a decrease of 10% or more from the predicted peak flow reading; (b) a sudden change in weather, including a sharp decrease in barometric pressure, sudden gusts of wind, a large change in humidity, etc.; (c) failure to adhere to medication instructions; and (d) strong exposure to other stimuli known to precipitate a given patient's asthma. The more the patient knows about the triggers of asthma, the greater the probability that an attack can be avoided. Thus, there is a need both to know precipitants of asthma and the self-monitoring of these stimuli if and when they appear in the environment.

Principle X: Through conditioning, antecedents can come to elicit automatic responses that are often emotional.

Because of previous experiences, there are patients who, when they begin to experience asthma, become frightened. This usually indicates that the fear has somehow become conditioned to attacks. There are a number of ways the patient can learn to manage such behaviors: First, the patient may wish to describe his or her feelings with the instructors of Asthma Self-Management. They will not only provide useful suggestions, but they will discuss treatment options with the patient. Second, the patient can treat him/herself through self-application of systematic desensitization (Wolpe, 1958). Earlier, we discussed the use of this procedure in a step-by-step fashion. Finally, the patient might try the stress inoculation method described by Meichenbaum (1986). This can help manage future attacks. There are any number of effective ways to treat the fear that may accompany an asthma attack; for this reason, appropriate techniques are available to help learn more useful responses which can occur as a consequence of an asthma attack. In addition, learning how to relax during attacks, instead of experiencing an emotional response, will permit more effective performance whatever steps are required to help bring a flare-up under control. There is no reason why fear, panic, or another type of emotional reaction should interfere with the management of asthma.

Principle XI: Many behaviors are learned by observing how other patients respond to their asthma. The patient can learn to imitate the skills which seem to help them manage their attacks.

We noted earlier that a great number of self-management skills can be learned by observing how other patients respond to their asthma. If the patient is hospitalized during an attack, he or she should observe to see if there is any particular patient who seems to know how to help bring an episode under control. The patient may want to later imitate such behaviors when suffering asthma. In addition, many ways to cope with asthma will be learned from others in the group. Most have faced problems similar to those the patient has experienced; the patient should attempt to pick up what appear as the best approaches to the management of these problems. The patient will again want to incorporate any of these steps into his or her own management of future attacks. And, patients should not forget: **When they successfully use a new step and it helps bring asthma under control, they should always reinforce themselves! A patient has not only made a significant contribution to the control of asthma, but the patient has demonstrated that he or she can continue to hone and refine the self-management skills already known!**

COMMON REASONS WHY SELF-MANAGEMENT PROCEDURES FAIL

There are a number of reasons, some of which were suggested by Watson and Tharp (1989), as to why self-management procedures fail (Table 5:2). These factors include:

TABLE 5:2. REASONS WHY SELF-MANAGEMENT PROCEDURES FAIL

Lack of commitment.

Failure at self-observation.

Failure to use self-management techniques.

Disbelief that the self-management techniques will work.

Disbelief that goals can be attained.

Wavering of commitment.

No real desire to want to change.

Too much time and effort required.

Failure to reinforce successes.

Discouragement after some successes.

Other people discouraging use of techniques.

Failure to adjust plans to fit needs.

Failure to attempt specific behaviors in array of settings.

Lack of patience.

Failure to use self-management skills to both establish control
over asthma and build self-efficacy beliefs.

---

1. Lack of commitment.

Patients must commit themselves to learning and applying self-management skills to help manage their asthma. Without this commitment, it is unlikely that they will benefit from Asthma Self-Management. Commitment is especially necessary, particularly at the start of their participation, because it is the major source of motivation for patients. Later, most will develop other strategies for self-motivation, including self-reinforcement. All motivational tactics, however, stem from the initial commitment of the patient to learn and perform self-management skills to help control his or her asthma.

2. Failure at self-observation.

    Without good observation, the patient may not reach the goals he or she has set. It is too easy for the patients to become inconsistent or impatient in monitoring their performance; the result may be the abandonment of self-management skills without giving themselves adequate opportunity to really try them out. In addition, self-observation forces the patient to think more clearly about the causes and results of performance. Keeping good records, even when initially unsuccessful at using self-management skills, can increase later chances for attaining success at performing these skills. It is important for the patients to be aware of the successes they have achieved and not just focus on any failures. The patient may not show dramatic changes in performance at first, but this is bound to change with continued effort.

3. Not using the technique.

    We have taught patients proven skills for the self-management of asthma. If a patient does not perform these skills when required for the control of attacks, then he or she cannot expect to see change. By performing these skills, however, the patient should not only become more proficient, but should see changes in the overall status of his or her asthma.

4. Disbelief that the techniques will help.

    The patient may believe that some of the skills we have asked him or her to perform really won't help in the event of an attack. If this is the case, then the patient is unlikely to perform the skills when an attack occurs. Skills in self-management and the attitudes towards these skills are inseparable; they go together like a hand and a glove. Without the belief that a difference really can be made in the control of asthma, self-management skills are unlikely to be performed. And, without practice at performing these skills, belief that a difference really can be made is not apt to be developed.

5. Disbelief that goals set can be attained.

    Bandura (1977) observed that one's belief that one can cope with a problem affects how hard one tries to overcome it and, in turn, affects success. Patients may lose what confidence they have if they either fail to perform self-management skills during attacks or only focus on failures. Patients must give themselves the chance to learn and perform these skills; with practice, confidence and belief that they will be successful will increase. **Each patient owes this to himself or herself!**

6. Wavering of commitment.

    No matter their initial commitment to learn and practice self-management skills, most patients occasionally waver in their commitment. The reason usually has to do with their asthma; it may worsen or they may suffer a severe attack even though they have taken every step to prevent such outcomes. For this reason, those involved with Asthma Self-Management, participants and staff members alike, must always be aware of the potential for a wavering of commitment or a weakening of motivation by patients. It should be explained that the severity of asthma often varies independently of the best actions of patients and their physicians; patients, in turn, must always be cognizant of this fact and make every effort to control as much as they can about their asthma. In the long run, they will realize that their commitment to learning and performance self-management skills was justified.

7. No real desire to want to change.

> We doubt that this is a factor with most of the patients involved in Asthma Self-Management: Patients will not do all that is asked if they do not want to learn and perform self-management skills to help control their asthma. There may be times when motivation for performing self-management skills can be weak; this sometimes occurs when an occasional patient comes to recognize that their control over their asthma destroys any secondary gain they may receive for being sick. We did not, fortunately, encounter any patients who would fall into this category in developing and evaluating Asthma Self-Management. It can happen, however. For this reason, it should be repeatedly stressed that **the patient, and only the patient, will be the major beneficiary of his or her efforts.**

8. Too much time and effort required.

> There may be periods of time when participating in Asthma Self-Management seems almost impossible to the patient. Factors preventing participation can include other serious health problems or difficult family problems. We recognize such problems occur and can be an impediment in participating in the program. However, the patient should not use this as an excuse for either failure to be involved in Asthma Self-Management or for not performing the self-management skills we have taught. They do require time and effort on the patient's part. However, performance of these skills can save considerable time and effort in the long run: They may prevent the patient's asthma from becoming more severe and requiring more intensive treatment, such as hospitalization, to be controlled.

9. Failure to reinforce success.

> Patients are reinforced for their performance throughout Asthma Self-Management. This generally takes the form of social reinforcement provided by other participants and staff members involved with the program. However, the most potent reinforcers are often the self-statements that patients make to themselves about their performance. Such statements as, "Hey, I did a nice job in controlling that attack!", strengthen the performance of self-management skills. Using self-statements as self-reinforcement helps develop what some call intrinsic reinforcement. This simply means that a major source of reinforcement is provided, contingent upon successful performance of self-management skills, by the individual; reinforcement here does not rest on recognition provided by others. It should always be emphasized that patients should reinforce themselves for performing self-management skills to help control their asthma. After awhile, they may take their successful performance for granted. This means that they have achieved a high level of intrinsic reinforcement and are confident about their ability to make a contribution to the management of their asthma.

10. Discouragement after some initial success.

It is not unusual for the patient to attain success when first beginning to perform self-management skills. This is a common finding. In most instances, this success will fuel future efforts on the patient's part. If any failure is encountered, however, the patient may want to give up. **The patient must not!** As Watson and Tharp (1989) explain:

> "Don't expect instant success. Be prepared to use a variety of techniques, and give them a chance to work. Expect to encounter obstacles, and use problem-solving techniques to overcome them" (p. 271).

11. Other people are discouraging use of the techniques.

Others, especially family members, may think it is silly of the patient to think that he or she can control asthma. They may think that all that is needed is willpower to manage attacks. The patient should not let others put temptations in the way that keep him or her from achieving the goal of making a contribution to the overall management of asthma. The patient should be assertive and proclaim the right to the best medical care that can be received for the control of asthma. This includes performance of self-management skills to help make a contribution to the control of asthma. **The patient should not be concerned about what others may tell him or her--after all, the patient is the one who will benefit from becoming an active partner with the physician in the management of asthma.**

12. Failure to adjust plans to fit needs.

A characteristic of asthma is its variability. This makes it difficult, if not impossible, to know beforehand how severe a given attack is apt to be. To help manage an episode, a patient must be flexible and prepared to manage whatever occurs during an attack. In most instances, the patient will manage his or her flare-up by following a prescribed step-wise treatment program; during more severe attacks, however, he or she may have to jump ahead in the treatment plan and request assistance from a physician or emergency room staff. Patients must adjust their plans to fit the needs of themselves and their asthma. Failure to adjust plans could result in the worsening of an episode from mild to severe. A repeated theme of Asthma Self-Management is that the patients learn to recognize their needs and make whatever adjustments are necessary in order to manage their asthma.

13. Failure to attempt specific behaviors in an array of settings.

Once patients learn to help manage their asthma at home, they will want to apply these same skills to help control attacks that occur in other settings, e.g., at work or school. Patients learn specific self-management skills; the value of these skills rests upon their being applied in whatever setting a patient is in when he or she suffers an attack. Applying self-management skills across settings increases the generalization of the program, as well as increasing the self-confidence of patients in their ability to contribute to the management of their asthma. Thus, it must always be emphasized that the patient apply the self-management skills they have acquired no matter what setting they are in. Only through this successful performance will they achieve full benefit of asthma self-management.

14. Lack of patience.

Let's face it: We all lack patience at one time or another. Patients with asthma are no different; if anything, they probably are more enduring in managing their disorder than we might be. Establishing control over asthma requires as much patience as can be generated by any patient. The intermittency, variability, and reversibility of the disorder, in and of themselves, try everyone's patience. The problem becomes even more pronounced, however, when there is a worsening of an attack despite everyone, including the patient, doing everything correctly. The patient must understand this outcome will eventually occur and not lose faith in his or her ability to apply self-management skills to make a contribution to the control of his or her asthma. Reiterating the need for patience can never be emphasized too strongly in teaching and reinforcing patients for assisting in the management of their asthma.

15. Failure to use self-management skills both to establish control over asthma and to build self-efficacy beliefs.

Failure to use self-management skills and to acquire a belief in their ability to help manage asthma will, in the long run, defeat any attempt to teach the skills taught in Asthma Self-Management. There is little likelihood that patients will build self-efficacy in their own abilities without performing self-management skills to help manage their asthma. Thus, there is the need to constantly remind the patient to apply self-management skills to help control his or her asthma; this motif is woven throughout the entire program.

RELAPSE PREVENTION

Watson and Tharp (1989) have several suggestions for preventing relapses in the use of self-management procedures. Those relevant to the self-management of asthma include:

1. Preparing for high risk situations.

If there is a seasonal component to asthma, the patient will want to prepare for this by being certain he or she can perform the self-management skills needed before they must be performed. The patient should be aware of environmental factors that can change and trigger asthma. The patient should also be aware of other factors, such as emotional distress, conflicts, or social pressures, that can influence the likelihood of successfully using self-management skills to help alleviate asthma. Being prepared for high risk situations can help the patient be successful at achieving the goals that have been set by participating in Asthma Self-Management.

2. Coping with high risk situations.

We have taught a number of techniques for coping with high risk situations. Those to be emphasized include: (a) deep muscle relaxation; (b) imagery; (c) self-instructions; (d) self-reinforcement; and (e) problem-solving skills. The patient should bring the entire array of self-management skills to help cope with high risk situations; this is the reason, after all, why the patient has been taught to perform such skills.

3. Putting on the brakes: Stopping lapses from becoming relapses.

We all have lapses in the self-management skills we perform, whether they be in controlling asthma or in managing our weight. What is important is that a lapse is not permitted to develop into a major relapse. This can be prevented by performing the coping skills described earlier. In addition, the patient can increase self-monitoring of behavior so as to take advantage of any cues or changes which will permit him or her to introduce self-management skills earlier in the attack. Lapses are failures on our part; as such, we can learn from our mistakes and avoid similar problems in the future.

Goleman (1988) notes that such lapses provide learning opportunities for patients. He notes several coping techniques that can be used for such lapses. These include having the patient: (a) treat the slip as an emergency that requires immediate action on his or her part, such as reviewing the self-management skills so that he or she is prepared to perform them during his or her next attack; (b) accept the fact that a slip is not a relapse, but only a temporary lapse from performing self-management skills; (c) renew his or her commitment to performing self- management skills to help control future attacks; (d) review his or her actions so that they will not be repeated in the future; (e) make an immediate plan for recovery by reviewing self-management techniques; and (f) ask for additional help if necessary. The key to success in the use of self-management skills is not only using them to help control asthma, but in keeping from relapsing and permitting the skills to extinguish.

PUTTING EVERYTHING TOGETHER

In her book, Borysenko (1988) lists 12 reminders for using psychological procedures to cope with physical disorders. Many of these reminders are of relevance to the self-management of asthma.

1. While you cannot control the external circumstances of your life, you can control your reaction to them.

We have stressed that there are many factors affecting asthma over which the patient will never establish control. However, it can be determined how the patient is going to react to asthma. The purpose of Asthma Self-Management is to teach the patient how to react to attacks; it provides him or her with a potent tool to make a significant contribution to the overall management of respiratory distress.

2. Optimal health is the result of both physical and mental factors.

We have emphasized the interaction that takes place between asthma and performance. We believe that the best way to make a contribution to the control of asthma is to consistently perform self-management skills. The strength of the interaction between asthma and performance will strengthen with practice. The beliefs patients have in their own ability will also increase. The result should be optimal health.

3. You should think of yourself as basically healthy.

    A number of years ago, Creer, Renne, and Christian (1976) pointed out that patients
    with asthma were healthy much of the time. It was only during attacks when this was not
    the case. We believe this attitude has more impact on the asthmatic patient than anyone:
    If patients think of themselves as basically healthy with only a problem they have to make
    allowances for--asthma--they will have a much better concept of themselves than if
    they basically think of themselves as sick. Thinking of themselves as healthy generates
    not only more confidence that the patients can help control asthma, but it expands the
    horizon with respect to the lifestyle patients want to adopt for themselves and their
    families.

4. Things change; change is the only constant in your life.

    There are times when self-management skills will not need to be performed to the
    degree that they will at other times. The patient needs always to be aware that things
    change. By learning and performing self-management skills, we believe that the patient
    will be much more capable of coping with asthma. At the same time, we believe the
    patient will be more ready to take advantage of the challenges presented by the changes
    that inevitably occur in life.

5. Your beliefs are extremely powerful.

    To a considerable degree, whether or not performance of self-management skills to
    help control asthma is successful is a function of the beliefs the patient has that such
    techniques are useful in achieving this goal. Patients must believe in themselves and in
    their ability to help control asthma. We believe that such attitudes will emerge and grow
    with sustained effort on the patient's part. If the patient always practices
    self-management skills when he or she needs to, the patient should be able to make a
    major contribution to the overall control of asthma.

6. The only escape from stress, fear, and doubt is to confront them directly and see them for
    what they really are.

    There is no way to hide from the stress that may be due to asthma. Trying to hide can
    only strengthen the fears of confronting reactions such as stress. The patient should try
    never to feel helpless. We believe that the patient possesses a powerful technology for
    changing reactions to asthma through the performance of self-management skills.

7. Emotions fall into two broad categories: Fear and love.

    We all know the fear of being unable to breathe; there is no need to expand upon this
    category. The love category is associated with openness and a sense of relaxing and letting
    go. Combining love with other self-management skills permits patients to expand the
    confidence they have in themselves. The latter, after all, is a form of healthy love that
    can only benefit the patient in the future.

8. Would you rather be right or would you rather experience peace?

   Always recognize self-worth and how to increase it. The patient need never to defend performance of self-management skills to anyone as "right." They are important because their performance will provide the patient with both better health and greater peace of mind.

9. Accept yourself as you are.

   The patient may never be the asthma-free, healthy person he or she once was, but he or she can certainly make the effort to become the healthiest asthmatic individual in the world. The patient knows what to do to achieve this goal; it is up to the patient to perform the necessary skills to achieve this aim.

10. Practice letting go.

    Asthma can make anyone, including the patient and members of the family, uptight. The patient should try and let go by performing the skills that have been taught. Once the patient feels confident with the performance of these skills, he or she and the family should think of other ways to let go and become involved in other activities that can do nothing but bring satisfaction to all family members, including the patient.

11. Stay open to life's teachings.

    What we have taught in Asthma Self-Management is but a beginning. With experience at performing self-management skills, the patient can see how these skills can be used to open up to new opportunities and experiences.

12. Be patient.

    We did not teach self-management skills in one day. We also do not expect that these skills will be performed perfectly the first time they are tried. However, the patient should be patient with him/herself and give him/herself the opportunity to perfect the performance. There is no reason why the patient cannot achieve this goal.

References

Bandura, A. (1977). Self-efficacy: Toward a unifying theory of behavioral change. Psychological Review, 84, 191-215.

Borysenko, J. (1988). Minding the body, mending the mind. New York: Bantam Books.

Creer, T. L., Renne, C. M., & Christian, W. P. (1976). Behavioral contributions to rehabilitation and childhood asthma. Rehabilitation Literature, 37, 226-232, 247.

Goleman, D. (1988, December 27). Breaking bad habits: New therapy focuses on the relapse. The New York Times, pp. 17-18.

Meichenbaum, D. (1986). Cognitive behavioral modification. In F. H. Kanfer & A. P. Goldstein (Eds.), Helping people change: A textbook of methods. 3rd edition (pp. 346-380). New York: Pergamon.

Watson, D. L., & Tharp, R. G. (1989). Self-directed behavior: Self-modification for personal adjustment. Fifth edition. Monterey, CA: Brooks/Cole Publishing Company.

Wolpe, J. (1958). Psychotherapy by reciprocal inhibition. Stanford, CA: Stanford University Press.

PSYCHOLOGICAL RESPONSES TO ASTHMA
VISUAL 5.1

Depressed feelings, low self-esteem, low self-worth

Low self-confidence, passivity

Anger

Panic

Fears and phobias

Secondary gain

FEAR: CAN ASTHMA BE FATAL?

VISUAL 5.2

INCIDENCE (quite rare)

.5 per 100,000 patients

On the rise?

-air quality

-better diagnosis

-increased severity of asthma in population

-increased prevalence of asthma

-inaccurate autopsies (i.e., over reporting)

PATIENT FACTORS

Disregard of symptoms

Delay in seeking help

Inappropriate self-care

-poor medication compliance

-use of only over-the-counter meds

-reliance on inhaled bronchodilators

Depression or psychosis; not related to asthma

(very rare)

Medical Care Factors

Disregard of symptoms

Delay in treating case

Inadequate monitoring of lung function and/or

blood gases

Sedation

Toxic dose of theophylline or other xanthine

Failure to use artificial ventilation

RESPONSES OF FAMILY AND FRIENDS

VISUAL 5.3

Doubts and accusations

Panic, fear

Shame, guilt, avoidance

Resentment, jealousy

Overprotectiveness

LIFE STYLE CHANGES
VISUAL 5.4

Becoming a homebody

Avoiding physical exercise

An asthma centered lifestyle

PHYSICAL CHANGES
VISUAL 5.5

FATIGUE

SLEEP DISTURBANCE

DECREASED PHYSICAL STAMINA

INCREASED SUSCEPTIBILITY TO INFECTION

SHAKINESS, NAUSEA, GASTROINTESTINAL
    PROBLEMS

ECONOMIC COSTS OF ASTHMA

VISUAL 5.6

DIRECT COSTS
   Physician Visits
   Medications
   Lab Work
   Hospitalizations

INDIRECT COSTS
   Transportation
   Income loss
   Asthma aids (hypoallergenic linens &pillows,
        humidifiers, etc.)

SOLVED PROBLEMS EXERCISE
VISUAL 5.7

(1) <u>S</u>tate the problem.	
(2) <u>O</u>utline the problem.	

(3)<u>L</u>ist solutions.
  a.
	(4)<u>V</u>iew the consequences.
	  +

	-
b.	+
	-
c.	+
	-
d.	+
	-
e.	+
	-
f.	+
	-
(5)<u>E</u>xecute your solution.	
(6)<u>D</u>etermine if solution is effective.	

SESSION SIX
PROBLEM SOLVING

GOALS
1. To finish presenting an overview of the consequences of asthma.
2. To introduce assertiveness training.
3. To educate patients about selecting a physician.
4. To conduct group problem solving.

EQUIPMENT
Name tags.
Paper and pencils for all participants.
Overhead projector or slide projector.

SUPPLIES
Coffee, tea, snacks, or light lunch.

SESSION SIX OUTLINE

TOPIC/ ACTIVITY	REQUIRED MATERIAL	APPROXIMATE TIME ALLOWED
Welcome & salutations	Name tags	5 minutes
Questions about prior sessions/ readings		10 minutes
Review SOLVED Problems worksheets		15 minutes
Consequences of asthma (cont.)	See Session 5 (Visuals 5.1-5.6)	as needed
SOLVE Feelings	Solve Feelings Worksheet, Visual 6.1	10 minutes
Assertiveness skills	Visual 6.2	10 minutes
Selecting a physician	Visual 6.3	10 minutes
Open discussion		10 minutes
Homework	Common Asthma Problems Checklist; SOLVED Problems; (Visual 6.4) SOLVE Feelings; (Visual 6.5) review all chapters	10 minutes

SESSION SIX TEACHING NOTES

Welcome and Salutations

Provide a name tag to each participant. Allow some time for small talk among group members prior to introducing the session material.

Questions About Prior Sessions/Readings

Allow the group to ask questions about material covered earlier in the program.

Review SOLVED Problems worksheets

Encourage the participants to share their problem-solving efforts, including both failures and successes, with the group. Reward all efforts with praise. Attempt to draw out participants' collective wisdom in solving asthma-related problems; the group will undoubtedly share some common problems. Allow the group to do as much of the problem solving as they can without leader feedback. Learning to generate potential solutions is more important than providing each participant with the one or two **best** solutions to their problem. Therefore, allow the group to generate several solutions before offering the obvious solution they may have missed.

Consequences of Asthma (continued from Session 5)

Resume the discussion of asthma consequences started in Session 5. The consequences of asthma have been divided into five major categories: psychological responses, responses of family and friends, lifestyles alterations, physical changes, and economic costs. Allow the group to generate as many consequences and solutions as possible before providing missing information. Welcome suggestions by participants and try to stimulate discussion and elicit innovative ways to deal with these problems. (See Visuals 5.1-5.6.)

SOLVE Feelings

The SOLVE Feelings exercise, a variation on the SOLVED Problems handout, is provided to help group members develop self-management strategies for working with troublesome thoughts and feelings. Introduce an example exercise to the group before breaking into small groups of 3 or 4 to practice the exercise. Ideally, at least one leader will be assigned to each small group. If time remains, the entire group can discuss different problem-solving plans that were generated. The SOLVE Feelings exercise can be continued in Session 7.

Assertiveness Skills

Review the importance of assertiveness in managing asthma and daily living. The Session 6 Background Readings and Chapter 8 in the client guide present overviews of this area. An effective method for covering this material is to allow your patients to generate definitions for the behaviors listed in Visual 6.2 and then role play specific problem situations involving use of the medical system, in families, at work, etc.

Selecting a Physician

Ask the group to generate the important things to consider when selecting a physician to treat asthma. The group-generated list can be supplemented with a discussion of the points in Visual 6.3.

Open Discussion

Allow time for open discussion prior to introducing the homework assignment.

Homework

Emphasize the difference between the acquisition of asthma knowledge and the performance of self-management skills. Homework assignments are designed to help individuals apply the knowledge they have gained and to begin using critical self-management skills. It is important to initiate a discussion of problems that patients may anticipate when completing the homework assignments.

This week's homework assignment is to complete a SOLVED Problems or SOLVE Feelings exercise, and to apply solutions to at least one asthma-related problem. Part of Session 7 will be used to discuss people's experiences with problem solving. Clients should also review the entire manual or read any chapters they have skipped; they will have an opportunity in the next session to ask questions about the material.

SESSION SIX BACKGROUND READING

BEING ASSERTIVE

Throughout these sessions, we have discussed patient rights as health care consumers. To obtain the services to which the patient is entitled, he or she needs to be assertive. This term, according to Alberti and Emmons (1986), is defined in the following manner:

> Assertive behavior promotes equality in human relationships, enabling us to act in our own best interests, to stand up for ourselves without undue anxiety, to express honest feelings comfortably, to exercise personal rights without denying the rights of others (p. 7).

There are key elements to this definition for the patient with asthma:

To promote equality in human relations means to put yourself on equal footing with your physician and other members of the medical staff. This makes it possible for everyone to gain and for no one to lose.

To act in your own best interests refers to your ability to make certain decisions about your asthma and to become a partner in the management of the disorder. It does not mean that you abandon any treatment plans prescribed for you without consulting your physician, but that you discuss any misgivings or concerns that you may have about the recommended treatment.

To stand up for yourself involves your expressing yourself about your asthma and its management. If you do not understand why you have been asked to follow a particular regimen, ask questions. Remember that there are no dumb questions.

To express feelings honestly and comfortably means the ability to express whatever feelings or thoughts you have about your asthma and its treatment to your physician. If you sometimes disagree with what is asked of you, don't hesitate to express your feelings in an attempt to resolve the matter.

To exercise personal rights refers to your ability to act competently as a health care consumer and to enhance your role as a partner with your physician in the treatment of your asthma.

To not deny the rights of others is to be able to achieve all of these personal expressions without unfair criticism of others, without hurtful behavior towards others, without name-calling, without intimidation, without manipulation, without controlling others.

Alberti and Emmons (1986) suggested steps for increasing assertiveness (Table 6:1).

TABLE 6:1. TEN CHARACTERISTICS REQUIRED TO ACHIEVE ASSERTIVE BEHAVIOR

(Suggested by Alberti & Emmons, 1986)

1. Self-expression;
2. Respect for the rights of others;
3. Honesty;
4. Direct and firm communication;
5. Equalizing through benefiting both the patient and the relationship with the physician and other medical personnel;
6. Verbal communication, including expressing the content of the message that one wishes to convey;
7. Nonverbal consistency, including the enhancement of the style of the message through eye contact, voice, posture, facial expression, gestures, distance, timing, fluency, and listening;
8. Appropriate behavior for the physician and the situation;
9. Socially responsible; and
10. Recognition that these skills are learned, not inborn.

If we apply them to asthmatic patients, these steps can be adapted in the following manner:

STEP I: OBSERVE OWN BEHAVIOR

The patient must keep a personal log to insure that he or she is assertive enough when concerned with asthma and its treatment.

STEP II: KEEP TRACK OF ASSERTIVENESS

In the same manner that he or she tracks and monitors certain aspects of asthma, the patient should log his or her own assertiveness for a week or so. Each day, the patient should record information about situations in which he or she responded assertively, as well as those past situations when he or she should have been assertive but was not. The patient should be certain to be systematic and honest with himself or herself.

STEP III: SET REALISTIC GOALS

The patient should select particular targets for himself or herself in being assertive. He or she should start with a small, low-risk step to maximize chances of success. Self-monitoring asthma-related behaviors is a good place to start.

STEP IV: CONCENTRATE ON A PARTICULAR SITUATION

Using imagery, the patient will want to visualize how he or she hopes to handle an upcoming visit with the physician or other medical staff. The patient should be certain to know the questions or comments he or she wishes to make and should visually imagine verbalizing such remarks.

STEP V: REVIEW RESPONSES

Since the patient is keeping data on his or her assertiveness, the patient should occasionally review this information. Situations that occurred and how they were handled should be noted . If the patient was not assertive in discussing an asthma regimen, he or she should plan to be so in future situations that require such a response; if the patient was assertive, he or she should reinforce himself or herself for the behavior.

STEP VI: OBSERVE AN EFFECTIVE MODEL

The patient may desire to watch how others respond to similar situations. The patient should observe how other patients or staff members respond to the physician; much can be learned from such observations.

STEP VII: CONSIDER ALTERNATIVE RESPONSES

Various ways to be assertive in a given situation should be considered. There is usually more than a single way to manage these circumstances. The patient will want to review all possible alternatives to decide the best response he or she can make under such a situation.

STEP VIII: IMAGINE HANDLING THE SITUATION

Through the magic of imagery, the patient should close the eyes and imagine how to handle a given situation. He or she will want to be both assertive and natural in the responses. Ways of coping through imagery should be developed; at the same time, this will permit the patient to dissolve any blocks that could occur.

STEP IX: PRACTICE POSITIVE THOUGHTS

The patient should develop a list of several positive statements that can be made to him/herself that are related to a given situation. These statements should be practiced often.

STEP X: GET HELP IF NEEDED

STEP XI: TRY IT OUT

After the patient has examined personal behavior, considered alternatives, observed an appropriate model, and practiced positive thoughts, he or she should try out new ways of dealing with the problem situation. This may entail that several of the steps presented in this discussion be repeated. The patient may also wish to role play particular situations either by himself or herself or with the assistance of a friend or family member.

STEP XII: GET FEEDBACK

This involves repeating Step V with emphasis upon the positive aspects of behavior. The patient should know both the strengths and weaknesses in his or her performance.

STEP XIII: BEHAVIOR SHAPING

The patient should repeat whatever steps are necessary to gradually shape behavior to approximate that which has been established as the target goal. This should be done until the patient feels comfortable with what he or she is doing.

STEP XIV: THE REAL TEST

The patient should now be ready to tackle the real world. Moving from intention to performance--being assertive with yourself--may be the most important step of all for the asthmatic patient.

STEP XV: FURTHER READING

This means that the procedures that help develop desired behaviors should be repeated for other specific situations that give trouble.

STEP XVI: SOCIAL REINFORCEMENT

The final step in being assertive is that the need for on-going support and rewards be understood. A system of rewards in the environment should be set up, and the patient should not fail to reinforce himself or herself when he or she has been assertive. Later, the patient will use self-statements to reinforce his or her behavior.

WHAT TO LOOK FOR IN SELECTING A PHYSICIAN AND MEDICAL PRACTICE

CHOICES IN OFFICE PROCEDURES

There are a number of important considerations a patient should review before selecting a physician or medical practice. Those questions that an asthmatic patient may ask of himself or herself include:

1. Is there a printed schedule of all fees for office visits, procedures, and tests? Does the office provide itemized bills? What is the system used with respect to billing insurance companies?

2. Are there posted hours as to when the physician can be reached during the week? Does the physician note arrangements he or she has made for weekend coverage? Where do patients go if the physician is out of town and unavailable to them?

3. Can appointments be scheduled with minimal waiting? Can longer appointments be scheduled when there are questions of the physician regarding either a patient's asthma or treatment? Will the physician promptly return any telephone calls made to his or her office?

4. Will the physician facilitate obtaining medical and hospital records if they are needed? Will the physician or members of his/her office staff provide copies of any test results?

5. Is the office staffed with competent professionals who are knowledgeable about asthma and its treatment? Does the physician employ a physician's assistant or nurse with a background in asthma or pulmonary diseases? Are other members of the office staff, such as laboratory workers, competent at their work? The latter two questions are important because there may be types of treatment which they will administer to patients for their asthma.

6. When patients go on vacation, can they obtain a letter from the physician as to how their asthma should be treated in the event an attack is suffered? This should include a brief description of asthma and how it has been successfully managed in the past. Be certain that the physician requests that he or she be contacted in the event that attending physicians who treat attacks require additional information.

7. Is there an established system within the office to provide refills of prescribed medications, particularly if the physician is out of town? It is better not to be in this situation, but patients may unexpectedly run out of a medication (particularly one dispensed by a nebulizer) during an attack; hence the concern.

CHOICES IN DIAGNOSTIC PROCEDURES AND TREATMENT

1. Will the physician explain the purpose of all diagnostic testing done to verify asthma and its causes? Will he or she explain specific tests, e.g., skin testing, or pulmonary function tests, e.g. FEV-1?

2. Will the physician provide the patient with a prognosis about his or her condition?

3. Will the physician discuss treatment and medication options for asthma by describing these options in terms that are understandable to the patient? The options include: (a) the purpose of each treatment, particularly the treatment of choice; (b) the potential risks of the latter treatment; (c) the potential side-effects that might reasonably be expected with any medications; (d) the costs of the treatment of choice, as well as any options for reducing costs if this is possible; (e) the length of time to be expected to receive any given treatment; and (f) any potential interactions of medication with foods, other medications, etc.

4. Will the physician or a member of his or her staff demonstrate how to take medications as instructed? This is particularly required when nebulized medications are prescribed.

5. What are the qualifications of the physician to perform the proposed diagnostic measures or treatments? Does the patient feel it would be better to consult with a specialist in asthma such as an allergist or chest physician?

6. Does the physician post his or her credentials on the walls of his or her office? Important documents that should be readily available for inspection include: (a) graduation diplomas from colleges and medical schools; (b) evidence of specialized training as an intern or resident; (c) evidence of completion of workshops on asthma or other respiratory diseases; and (d) a valid license to practice medicine in the state.

7. Will the physician provide information about organizations, such as the American Lung Association, which publish materials on asthma? Are there materials from these and other organizations concerned with asthma in the physicians's waiting room?

8. Before initiating any treatment or before altering the treatment being received, will the physician explain the changes and receive agreement before they are initiated?

PERSONAL QUALITIES OF COMPETENT PHYSICIANS (including suggestions by Manning and DeBakey, 1987)

We all have qualities that we wish to see in our personal physician. We want someone who not only understands our physical problems, but who can listen to us in a warm and genuine manner. He or she can also provide us with the sympathy that is often as important as medicine in helping us overcome pain and physical difficulties. All of us, including those with asthma, search for such physicians. Manning and DeBakey (1987) recently reviewed the characteristics of physicians who were considered to be the best by their colleagues. The personal qualities found by Manning and DeBakey (1987) are certain to be among those we all look for in finding our own personal physician.

I.   PERSONALITY CHARACTERISTICS INCLUDE:

A.   **Personal confidence, self-respect, and pride in working with patients.**
Physicians considered as highly competent are not only confident, but they take pride in their work. Confidence can be contagious: If the physician seems confident about what he or she is doing, the patient will believe in the physician.

B.   **Enjoyment in working as a physician.** We all sense whether people enjoy their work (certainly, we know the degree of satisfaction and pleasure we receive from our employment!). Physicians are no different. Some truly enjoy helping solve the complex puzzle presented by asthma and those afflicted by the disorder. Those are the physicians that should be sought out by those with asthma.

C.   **Curiosity.** Most prominent physicians believe, according to Manning and DeBakey (1987), that an insatiable curiosity was innate or established in early childhood. At the same time, all recognized the need to continually nourish curiosity. Many physicians are not satisfied with an immediate or superficial answer, but want to go beyond this option to be certain their diagnosis and treatment regimen are the best available.

D.   **Discipline, diligence, and determination.** All competent physicians recognize the need for lifetime learning. This may take the form of setting aside times to read current journals or keeping reprint files of articles pertaining to their interests. Many physicians believe that writing an occasional article, even in the midst of a busy practice, provides them with a sense of discipline in keeping up with their interests.

E. **Compassion and a sense of service.** This was best stated by Sir Berkeley Moyihan (quoted in Manning & DeBakey, 1987, p. 6):

> "A patient can offer you no higher tribute than to entrust you with his life and health, and, by implication, with the happiness of all his family. To be worthy of such trust we must submit for a lifetime to the constant discipline of unwearied effort in the search of knowledge; and of most reverent devotion to every detail in every operation that we perform."

To many physicians, compassion is regarded as an important component of competence.

F. **Develops strong patient/physician relationship.** Repeatedly throughout their book, Manning and DeBakey (1987) note that good physicians are good listeners. They take the time to listen to their patients in an atmosphere characterized by unrushed attention. They ask thoughtful questions because they recognize that correct answers can only be reached through information supplied by the patients. They want their patients to be their partners in the management of the patients' diseases and discomfort. Physicians supplied what answers they could, but were willing to admit that they did not have answers for all questions. Rather than damage the patient/physician relationship, the latter approach has often been cited by patients as a strength of their physician.

G. **Were competent physicians.** The book by Manning and DeBakey (1987) is based upon interviews with many of the most prominent physicians practicing in the United States. All were highly competent physicians. A number of participants in asthma self-management programs have stated that they believe that knowledge and experience are the two qualities they most search for in a physician. They believe this quality is even more important that the "bedside" manners of their physician. As one participant put it, "My doctor could use lessons in his bedside manners, but I have no doubts about his competence. In the long run, this is what matters to me."

II. LEARNING FROM EXPERIENCE

William Osler is quoted by Manning & DeBakey (1987, p. 6):

> "To study the phenomena of disease without books is to sail an uncharted sea, while to study books without patients is not to go to sea at all."

Those physicians who learn from their experience appear to engage in the following practices:

A. **Obtain firsthand experiences.**

Competent physicians make every effort to gain experiences with the diseases and disorders they are apt to diagnose and treat. They are also credited with:

1. Carefully monitoring their own practice as it often is the most fruitful education for a profession.

2. Displaying self-directed learning to increase his or her knowledge through an analysis of his or her practice.

3. Making the most of their situations; even cases that appear routine to the average physician offer opportunities for learning to better physicians.

B. **Develop companionships in medicine.** The collegial network formed by physicians provides them with strong support for sharing experiences, knowledge, and inspiration in atmosphere that, while promoting fellowship, also promotes self-directed learning.

C. **Reduce reliance on memory.** Manning and DeBakey (1987) caution that acquiring knowledge when it is needed is more important than memorizing facts that may not be used for weeks or months. There is danger of knowledge that is unused. Manning and DeBakey again cite Whitehead (p.10) who stated:

> "Get your knowledge quickly, and then use it. If you can use it, you will retain it...Knowledge does not keep any better than fish."

D. **Frame the right questions.** Good physicians ask themselves questions, and then find the answers. They know what they know and what they do not know. As our ability to gather and store information has increased, increased emphasis has been placed on asking the best questions to take advantage of this information.

E. **Set priorities.** Formulating concrete and attainable goals not only enhances a physician's satisfaction, but improves his or her performance.

F. **Develop skills in reasoning and communication.** A number of the eminent physicians interviewed by Manning and DeBakey (1987) emphasized that they constantly were honing their skills of reasoning about problems and their solutions. Communicating these solutions to patients or to colleagues through writing was also a skill that was repeatedly stressed.

G. **Keep current.** Almost every physician interviewed by Manning and DeBakey (1987) described the importance of keeping up with their speciality. A number of techniques, ranging from establishing reprint files to using the computer, were suggested as ways in which physicians might self-educate themselves on current events. Presenting papers, attending medical conferences, or having consultants in on a regular basis were described as other techniques for keeping up to date with specialty knowledge. Guiding principles for reading were listed as:

1. Relating reading to experience.

2. Screening materials with respect to the physician's need, relevance, and validity.

3. Taking notes and making mental summaries.

4. Scheduling regular times for reading.

5. Following specific investigators known to be making significant contributions to the field.

6. Keeping new advances in historical perspective.

BEING A GOOD CONSUMER OF HEALTH CARE SERVICES

At one time or another we are all consumers of health care services. We are excellent consumers as indicated by the fact that almost 12% of our Gross National Product in the United States is devoted to health care services. While we may complain to ourselves about the type and quality of medical treatment we receive, we usually do nothing more about the situation. This is a mistake. We should consider the health care we receive in the same manner as any other purchase. After all, we are paying plenty for the privilege of receiving health and medical services. Thus, to be an effective health care consumer, the following suggestions are offered (Table 6:2):

TABLE 6:2. LEARNING TO BECOME AN EFFECTIVE HEALTH CARE CONSUMER

Learn to complain.

Never be angry when complaining.

Be confident of your ability to complain and eventual success.

Be knowledgeable about your complaint.

Know where to complain.

Begin at the source of your concern.

Be persistent.

Remember that it is in the best interest of your physician and
  other medical personnel to resolve your complaint.

---

1. **Complaining is an art.** The strategy you take with your mechanic probably won't work with your physician. Think out beforehand the tactics you are going to pursue if you have complaints about your medical treatment; jot them down and don't rely on memory. You likely will want to begin with a telephone call to your physician or comments during a regularly scheduled visit.

2. **Never be angry when you complain about medical treatment.** Being angry may work in some situations, but it will not be effective in complaining about medical treatment. Thus, if you are angry, wait until you have calmed down before taking any action. You never want to sound hostile. Your physician is more apt to listen to you if you remain calm.

3. **Be confident both of your right to complain and of your eventual success.**
   If you are timid at the outset, you are apt to be more frustrated than successful in pursuing your actions. You need to muster up all the confidence and self-beliefs that you can; if you do, you should be successful.

4. **Be knowledgeable about your complaint.** Know exactly what the problem is before initiating any action. Establishing the right tone for the initial salvo is important. Outline your complaint in a manner which allows you to make a thorough and systematic complaint. This should enhance the likelihood that you will succeed.

5. **Know where to complain.** If you are in a hospital setting, you may wish to contact the facility's patient representative. If in a clinic, you may wish to speak with an administrator or with your physician. You probably are not going to go far if you end up arguing with the clinic's receptionist.

6. **Begin at the source of your concern and go from there.** Usually, the matter will·be satisfied at the physician's office or clinic. However, if you feel your complaints have not been resolved, you can always contact the local medical society. In a hospital, you always have the option of working up through the administrative chain of command.

7. **Be persistent.** If you believe that your concerns have not been satisfactorily addressed, say so. Schedule extra time to talk with your physician during your next regularly scheduled visit. Everyone has the right to obtain the best available treatment for themselves and their families.

8. **Remember that it is probably as important to your physician and his or her staff as it is to you that your complaints are resolved.** Physicians want to provide the best service they can; after all, their livelihood is dependent upon providing quality treatment. Thus, they will usually go the extra step to be certain that your complaints are resolved.

WAYS TO ANTAGONIZE YOUR PHYSICIAN

There are a number of ways that a patient may, sometimes unwittingly, upset a physician. We have noted a few common complaints of physicians about their patients with asthma (Table 6:3).

TABLE 6:3. WAYS TO ANTAGONIZE YOUR PHYSICIAN

Ask for unnecessary medications or laboratory tests.

Be hostile, disrespectful, demeaning, or critical.

Be manipulative.

Arrive dirty, unkempt, and with poor hygiene.

Ask for new medications before they are developed or available.

Overestimate or underestimate the severity of your asthma.

Be untruthful.

Complain about the number of forms you are asked to complete.

Be unprepared for the meeting.

Be non-compliant with physician's instructions.

The patient may wish to review these patient behaviors to be certain that he or she does not perform them so as to inadvertently antagonize the physician.

1. **Patient wants unnecessary medications or laboratory tests.** The patient is more than welcome to ask questions of the physician regarding medications and laboratory tests. What is apt to arouse the physician is when the patient demands that he or she be given certain medications or receive additional testing when the physician does not believe this would benefit the patient in any way. These requests are not the same as the patient explaining to the physician that the medication being taken is not controlling the asthma or that the patient believes that he or she might be able to cut back on the dosage; it is the repeated request, in the absence of any firm data, that other medications be prescribed or additional tests conducted.

2. **Patient is hostile, disrespectful, demeaning, or critical.** Throughout this program, we have discussed how the patient can become a partner with the physician in the management of asthma. Becoming a partner does not mean, however, that the patient becomes hostile, disrespectful, demeaning, or unduly critical of his or her physician. What it means is that, through self-monitoring, the patient objectively observe his or her asthma. When the patient thinks that his or her partner, in this case the physician, would benefit from sharing this information, the patient passes it along. This should be done in a manner that is conducive to furthering the partnership with an introductory comment such as, "I thought you would like to know that..." This could be contrasted with, "I found out that my asthma medication doesn't seem to work. What the hell are you going to do about it?" While the latter would be indicative of assertiveness, it also

reflects hostility on the patient's part. There can be a fine line between being assertive and hostile, disrespectful, or demeaning. The patient should be certain to avoid crossing this line with the physician and other medical personnel.

3. **Patient is manipulative.** A number of physician complaints can be cataloged here, ranging from the patient's repeated interruptions to not listening to the physician's advice. All of this is not lost upon the physician, who begins to think it a waste of time in speaking with the patient. If, in the future, any instructions to the patient can be entrusted to a nurse, the physician will certainly try and direct patients this way. It is again important for the patient to remember that he or she is an ally with the physician in the treatment of asthma. This means that neither try and manipulate the situation, but that both cooperate and share responsibility for attempting to arrive at a satisfactory outcome--the control of a patient's asthma.

4. **Patient appears dirty, unkempt, and with poor hygiene.** No one, including most patients, likes to be around someone who is unkempt, smelly, and generally with poor hygiene. The patient doesn't like to be around such individuals, why should the physician? The patient should be certain to prepare for appointments by showing care about his or her appearance; this demeanor, in turn, will indicate to the physician that the patient is serious about his or her health.

5. **Patient wants new medications before they are developed.** This is a common complaint: Each time a medical or scientific breakthrough is announced, the patient believes that this represents an immediate cure for asthma. Such an attitude is certainly normal. However, the patient must remember that the average time between a basic discovery and applications that occur because of the discovery is approximately 25 years. Thus, any basic discovery today is not apt to help the patient immediately manage his or her asthma. More than likely, the physician, particularly if he or she is an allergist or pulmonary specialist, is aware of any new medications that may enter the market. If he or she believes that such drugs can help control asthma, it can almost be certain that they will be prescribed. If they are not prescribed, the patient can always ask the physician if he or she thinks a newly-approved medication would help the patient and his or her asthma.

6. **Patient overestimates or underestimates the severity of his or her asthma.** Physicians who treat asthma frequently note this vexing problem: While some patients overestimate the severity of their asthma, others underestimate its severity. In the former case, the patient may think that his or her asthma is debilitating when it actually is not. In this event, the patient may limit activities when it is not necessary to do so. The physician, plus the information the patient gathers on himself or herself, will provide a good barometer of the physical limits. On the other hand, the patient may be the type who underestimates the severity of his or her asthma. When this occurs, the patient may not take every effort to prevent or avoid attacks; this can take the form of unnecessary exposure to stimuli that can precipitate an attack, such as keeping a dog in the house when animal dander triggers an attack, or not taking medications as prescribed. In either case, the patient's behavior is reflective of his or her underestimating the severity of asthma.

7. **Patient is untruthful.** Physicians are not only upset when patients are untruthful in answering questions, but the patients' answers may lead to a mistake in the treatment. An example here would be the answer to the question, "Do you smoke?" If the answer is no when the patient actually does still smoke cigarettes, the physician can prescribe an incorrect dosage of medication for the patient. The result in this case could either be a lack of control over asthma or medication toxicity. When the patient is truthful, no matter what the question, the patient has helped fulfill his or her end of the partnership established with the physician. The physician is thus capable of being of greater assistance to the patient.

8. **Patient complains about number of forms to complete.** Like everyone else, physicians do not like to complete any more forms than required for their practice. There is not much the patient can do about this with the exception of avoiding any unnecessary duplication of effort on the part of the physician and the staff in completing such materials.

9. **Patient is unprepared for meeting.** When the patient is prepared for the meeting, such as bringing along a list of questions, everything goes smoother. If the patient is not prepared, the physician not only is unable to accurately assess the condition, but he or she can expect a number of telephone calls from the patient to clarify any instructions that were provided--questions about any side-effects of a treatment, etc. Thus, as the Boy Scouts say, be prepared.

10. **Patient is non-compliant with physician instructions.** It is doubtful that there is a behavior more upsetting to a physician than the patient's failure to comply with instructions. The doctor realizes that the patient is not going to be perfectly compliant; almost everyone misses a prescribed dose of medication sometimes. However, the physician has the right, as part of the partnership, to believe that the patient will make a conscious effort to comply with instructions. The physician can then maximally use his or her expertise to assist the patient; when the patient does not comply, this expertise is wasted. It is particularly upsetting to physicians to discover that the patient has not only failed to take medications as prescribed, but he or she has not even bothered to fill the prescription at a pharmacy. It is doubtful that the Asthma Self-Management participant will ever fall into this category--he or she would not be attending this course if this were the case--but the illustration does provide the reason why physicians can become so upset when patients fail to comply with medical instructions. The patient should always make an effort to comply with the physician's instructions as his or her part of the partnership agreement being forged with the physician.

PROBLEM SOLVING

Each day, we all make numerous decisions to solve problems so as to live better and happier lives. We have emphasized ways to make decisions and solve problems throughout Asthma Self-Management. What follows are other approaches suggested for problem solving; all incorporate decision-making skills. These skills can be used in conjunction with the self-management skills that have been taught to help control asthma and to live fuller, more meaningful lives.

There are no more important tasks than that we successfully solve the myriad array of problems we face each day. Many are relatively easy to solve; we may quickly decide whether we should take an umbrella with us if the weatherman suggests it will rain. Other problems, such as whether we should apply for a job in another state, require careful and prolonged consideration before we make our final decision. Solving problems is an individual matter. There are many of us who may be very good at solving problems; we all have acquaintances who seem to have an almost uncanny ability to solve problems. Most of us, however, may not be this fortunate; we may find it either difficult to solve problems of daily living or, just as importantly, we may doubt our ability at performing these tasks.

There are certain points about problem solving on which most experts agree: First, problem-solving skills can be taught. We can learn how to solve problems with appropriate training. Second, there are ways to avoid many of the problems we face. We have stressed avoiding asthma attacks because by achieving this goal, the patient will not have to experience the distress of an asthma attack. Third, we must be positive and not negative about solving problems. As emphasized earlier, the patient can learn to use positive thoughts to help manage asthma; he or she can also learn to use similar thoughts to manage the other non-asthma-related problems faced each day. Finally, we must concentrate on solving daily problems. They usually do not go away of their own accord; they also are not usually solved by not attending to their resolution. When the patient's attention wanes, he or she may wish to follow strategies taught in Asthma Self-Management: (a) slow down the actions; (b) relax and think through the alternatives to solving the problem; (c) visualize what are likely to be the consequences of the action; (d) do not let attention drift or, if it does, begin repeating this sequence of events; and, (e) select what appears to be the best solution for solving the particular problem. These exercises will help in not only solving asthma-related difficulties, but also the other problems faced each day. They can also be repeated when, as we are all prone to do, an incorrect decision is made in an attempt to solve a problem. That is just a part of life for everyone, although we believe we can teach how to improve problem-solving skills.

There are a number of approaches that can be taken to solve problems. We are going to highlight several suggested ways to make decisions and to solve problems.

IDEAL PROBLEM SOLVING

Bransford and Stein (1984) have described what they refer to as the **IDEAL** problem-solving model. The **IDEAL** is an acronym for the steps they believe are imperative to solve problems. The steps, as applied to asthma, are:

I = IDENTIFYING PROBLEMS.

> Before a problem can be solved, it must be identified. This calls for careful analysis of the situation and specifying the problem as precisely as possible. It is helpful if potential problems can be pinpointed before they occur. If the likelihood of an asthma attack can be predicted by performing some action, such as monitoring peak flow values, performing the act may permit the prevention of the episode.

D = DEFINING PROBLEMS.

The problem should be defined and represented as carefully as possible. Preciseness is imperative not only in defining a problem, but in communicating anything about it to others. This can also be of assistance with respect to overcoming any memory limitations, particularly if the problem is apt to take a period to resolve, such as occurs with chronic asthma.

E = EXPLORING ALTERNATIVE SOLUTIONS.

This highlights the significance of performing a systematic analysis of all the possible alternative solutions to a problem. All of the skills learned in Asthma Self-Management, including the use of the A-B-C's of breaking down a problem, should be used. Bransford and Stein (1984) suggest three general strategies for exploring alternative solutions; these are similar to other strategies taught participants.

1. **Break down a complex problem into simpler components if possible.** This will sometimes permit solving a complex or abstract problem by focusing on simpler, specific solutions; the theme has been stressed throughout the Asthma Self-Management program.

2. **Working backwards from the solution to the steps taken in arriving at this point can also be helpful.** This seems to be an especially appealing approach when there is a goal in mind, e.g., improved management of asthma, but the exact steps that need to be taken to reach this goal are not certain.

3. **Search for approaches others have taken to solve a similar problem.** If others have successfully solved such problems, there is no need to reinvent the wheel; solutions suggested by others for managing asthma may be more than adequate.

A = ACTING ON A PLAN.

In Asthma Self-Management, time has not only been spent in learning to identify problems, but in how to solve them. Now that such skills have been acquired, they must be performed on a regular basis in order to achieve the goal of the program, e.g., the management and control of asthma.

L = LOOKING AT THE EFFECTS.

Evaluation has been a cornerstone of Asthma Self-Management, ranging from the paper-and-pencil tests completed to the twice daily use of the peak flow meter. There may be other ways to evaluate performance; here, it is suggested to be creative and tailor the evaluation tactic to what is to be determined about the performance. Bransford and Stein (1984) identify three blocks which may interfere with the effort to be a creative problem solver:

1. One may experience tunnel vision and think of only one solution to a problem. This limits the opportunity to attempt to consider other, perhaps more appropriate, solutions. Tunnel vision can interfere with a patient receiving the most appropriate treatment for a given attack, particularly one that is of rapid onset.

2. Emotional reactions can interfere with attempts to solve problems. The use of deep muscle relaxation skills have been emphasized not only because we think they can help in the overall management of asthma attacks, but because they can help the patient keep calm and think through the steps that need to be performed to help control a flare-up.

3. We are all ignorant about the best possible ways to manage the day-to-day problems we face. By participating in Asthma Self-Management, the patient has acquired considerable knowledge and expertise about the management of asthma. It is now up to the patient not only to perform the skills that have been taught, but to become more skilled at taking such action. This will help overcome any ignorance the patient may feel about the contribution he or she can make towards the management of asthma.

PERSONAL PROBLEM SOLVING (PPS)

Mahoney (1979) has offered an approach to self-change. He suggests that more credit be given to skillpower over willpower; in other words, the skills the patient has learned for managing asthma are generally more important than willpower. At the risk of oversimplification, Mahoney (1979) suggests that the cause of a problem is always: (a) a situation; (b) a behavioral pattern; or (c) a thought pattern. We believe that we would be remiss if we did not add (d)--physical distress--to this list of problems. In many cases, it is a combination of these factors which creates the problem for the patient.

Mahoney (1979) advocates that what he refers to as Personal Problem Solving (PPS) be used. He believes that a person who is good at resolving personal problems is a good "personal scientist." A good personal scientist would consider the following stages of scientific inquiry:

S = SPECIFY THE GENERAL PROBLEM AREA.

> This suggests the asthmatic patient delineate the general problem area that he or she wishes to investigate as a scientist. Resolution of the problem could result in improved control over asthma.

C = COLLECT INFORMATION.

> This is self-explanatory; the patient may have already collected more information on himself or herself than he or she wishes to know!

I = IDENTIFY POSSIBLE CAUSES.

> This means that the patient identify the antecedent events that occurred prior to an attack. Looking at the A-B-Cs of a problem, emphasized throughout the program, can provide considerable information.

E = EXAMINE POSSIBLE SOLUTIONS.

As stressed throughout this discussion, it is important that the patient consider all possible solutions to any problem he or she faces. In managing asthma, this means that the patient will wish to consider all possible skills that might be performed to help bring an attack under control. Mahoney (1979) suggests four steps be taken in examining possible solutions: (a) know what the solutions are; (b) evaluate these solutions; (c) think of alternative ways of viewing the problem; and (d) try out alternative ways of solving a problem.

N = NARROW SOLUTIONS AND EXPERIMENT.

Mahoney (1979) suggests five questions that might be asked; these are relevant to patients with asthma.

1. Is my proposed solution realistic and will I be able to implement it?

2. Is it really likely to produce the results I want?

3. What obstacles have I overlooked?

4. Is the solution worse than the problem?

5. How might I revise my proposed solution to make it more successful?

   These are all questions the patient may wish to consider in narrowing and experimenting with potential solutions to a problem.

C = COMPARE THE PROGRESS.

Mahoney (1979) points out that one may wish to look for changes in four areas: (a) the **frequency** of the problem behavior; (b) the **intensity** of the experience; (c) the **duration** of the experience; and (d) the **patterning** of the experience.

E = EVALUATION.

In evaluating the success of the attempt to solve a problem, one might consider it from six basic views (Mahoney, 1979):

1. Avoid dichotomizing what was done as either a success or failure; nothing is usually a total success or a total failure. And, as we noted earlier in discussing negative thoughts, sometimes a negative thought can be turned into a positive solution.

2. Set sights on improvement, not total resolution. The patient may still suffer the same frequency of asthma attacks, but through self-management, they should become less severe.

3. A personal experiment is a failure only if it does not provide information. One learns something about oneself from any failure, including the inability to control an attack by oneself.

4. It is important that the patient not only accepts responsibility for his or her choices, but also appreciates the fact that what he or she does is affected both by asthma and by the level of self-management skills.

5. There are some problems that are solved only by acceptance. With asthma, there is no cure; the best the patient can provide is to make life easier for himself or herself. This achievement, in itself, is a major victory.

6. Professional assistance should be sought as a possible option if unable to solve a particular problem.

PACE/DESIGN

This two-stage approach was developed by Creer (1980) as a way to teach problem-solving skills to students. They are also applicable to patients with asthma. The two stages are:

P = POTENTIAL PROBLEM.

This may be any event--cognitive, behavioral, environmental, or physical--that is considered to be a problem by a patient. Asthma certainly qualifies as a problem according to this criterion.

A = ANALYZE PROBLEM.

This entails that one consider an analysis of the A-B-Cs--antecedents, presenting behavior, and consequences that follow the behavior.

C = COLLECT INFORMATION.

As has been done throughout participation in Asthma Self-Management by Adults, this involves observation and recording of aspects of performance.

E = EVALUATE INFORMATION.

This will permit a decision as to whether or not a problem actually exists and what to do about it. If the problem is not severe, one may wish to discontinue the efforts; if the problem is strong enough to warrant action, move on to **DESIGN**.

D = DEFINE PROBLEM OPERATIONALLY.

This approach insures that one will define the specific problem faced with; it also permits obtaining more accurate data regarding the problem.

E = ESTABLISH GOALS.

Here, specify what the goals of self-intervention are in approaching the problem.

S = SELECT INTERVENTION PROCEDURE.

This entails selection of a procedure according to whether the aim is to shape, increase, extend, maintain, restrict, or reduce skill required to change the problem.

I = INSTITUTE AND CARRY OUT PROCEDURE.

This involves that one: (a) determine baselines; (b) select evaluation system; (c) apply intervention procedures; (d) maintain skill change; and (e) establish generality of the change.

G = GATHER CORRELATED DATA.

This entails the assessment of any changes in other measures that occur as a consequence of intervention. An example would be a change that could occur in the amount of medication the patient requires for the control of asthma as a result of the performance of self-management skills.

N = NOTIFYING OTHERS.

This involves that the results obtained be shared with the physician and other health care personnel.

FIVE GENERAL STEPS FOR PROBLEM SOLVING

In what are likely the most referenced steps for problem solving, D'Zurilla and Goldfried (1971) outlined the following five steps for solving personal problems:

G = GENERAL ORIENTATION.

You are encouraged to recognize asthma-related problems and to realize that it is possible to deal with them by acting systematically rather than impulsively. You may be taught to recognize problems by being presented with common examples of them and/or by being asked to describe such situations that you have encountered in your own life.

P = PROBLEM DEFINITION.

By specifying the history of the asthma-related problem and the variables that seem to influence it, it is usually possible to define the problem more precisely.

G = GENERATION OF ALTERNATIVES.

Here, you are asked to "brainstorm" possible solutions. This permits you to generate as many potential solutions as possible, no matter how farfetched many may seem.

D = DECISION MAKING.

You are then asked to examine the alternatives carefully and eliminate those that are unacceptable. You should think of the likely effectiveness of any given solution, as well as the short-term and long-term consequences that are apt to result from such action. On the basis of these considerations, you should select the alternative that seems most likely to provide the optimal solution; you can then devise a plan for performing the skills required to reach this goal.

V = VERIFICATION.

Does your plan solve the problem when it is put into effect? Are you satisfied with the results? If you answer no to either of these questions, then you want to consider another alternative solution to your problem.

STAGES FOR DECISION MAKING

Wheeler and Janis (1980) describe five stages for making decisions:

STAGE I: Accepting the Challenge

Decision making begins when you are confronted with a challenge to your current course of action. You then either have the choice of accepting the challenge or ignoring it and bearing the consequences. What is important in this stage is whether the challenge of having asthma is great enough to warrant your making the effort to make an active decision about it.

STAGE II: Searching for Alternatives

When your current course of action is challenged, you should begin searching for alternatives. Effective decision makers accomplish two things in Stage II: (1) they thoroughly consider their goals and values relevant to a decision; and (2) they use this information to search carefully through a wide range of alternatives that have promise of achieving these goals (Wheeler & Janis, 1980). Little evaluation of alternatives should occur during this stage; evaluation will come later.

STAGE III: Evaluating Alternatives

During this stage, you carefully consider the advantages and disadvantages of each alternative. This may require considerable effort on your part; however, effective decision makers seek facts and forecasts from a wide variety of sources about the consequences of the alternatives they are considering. Patients with asthma also carefully weigh both the positive and negative aspects of each alternative; this permits them, at the end of Stage III, to have reached a tentative decision based on the information they have gathered (Wheeler & Janis, 1980).

STAGE IV: Becoming Committed

At this point, the final choice is made and you commit yourself to a new course of action. You may wish to re-examine all of the information you have gathered before you make such a commitment.

STAGE V: Adhering to the Decision

We hope that you have made the right choice and that everything will go as you plan. If it does not, then you must be prepared to deal with setbacks and failure by accepting the new challenge and returning to the beginning to start a new cycle presented by the five stages.

SELECTING ALTERNATIVES

Wheeler and Janis (1980) have suggested several rules for selecting alternatives; in many ways, these are also good rules to consider in making good decisions. They are:

RULE I: Do not evaluate at the beginning.

When a new adventure, such as participating in Asthma Self-Management, is started, one may be uncertain as to whether or not to continue. However, learning and performing self-management skills requires time and patience. For this reason, progress should not be evaluated until after having had an opportunity to actually use self-management skills. The same advice holds true for making other decisions: Rather than evaluate at the beginning, define the data that is to be collected in order to analyze progress. This information will later be of assistance in making any decision.

RULE II: Generate as many alternatives as possible.

We have described ways that one can generate as many alternative choices as possible. One may wish to: (a) brainstorm; (b) develop as many ideas as possible; (c) talk with others; and (d) throughout the entire process, attempt to keep emotions at a point where they do not interfere with decisions.

RULE III: Try to be original.

Rather than accept the tired and hackneyed ideas of others, think of new alternatives. The patient is likely the most knowledgeable expert with respect to all aspects of asthma. For this reason, he or she may have other ideas that can help control attacks. If so, the patient may want to discuss with the physician or other staff the possibility of including them in the self-management program.

RULE IV: Modify flawed alternatives.

If there is an alternative choice with flaws, one may want to rethink the choice. This can suggest ways to revamp the idea or to combine it with other alternatives.

RULE V: Ask other people.

When thinking of possible choices regarding asthma, the patient might wish to bounce some ideas off the physician or members of the project staff. The patient should go to those he or she trusts for advice if there is a need for assistance. The patient should remember, however, that they are merely giving their opinion; the decision as to what step to take is ultimately up to the patient.

RULE VI: Use contemplation as a source of ideas.

Generally, there is time to choose among alternatives before making a decision. If you have this luxury, take your time. Think of each decision that might be made and the likely consequence of that decision. This will permit some idea of what events will occur when a decision is made.

RULE VII: Avoid dichotomies.

Whenever faced with an either/or situation, one should try to take a broader view of the matter to see whether it is possible to arrive at other alternatives. This permits escape from a situation where there are but two choices to select between.

References

Alberti, R. E., & Emmons, M. L. (1986). <u>Your perfect right: A guide to assertive living</u>. San Luis Obispo, CA: Impact Publishers.

Bransford, J. D., & Stein, B. S. (1984). <u>The IDEAL problem solver: A guide for improving thinking, learning, and creativity</u>. New York: W. H. Freeman and Company.

Creer, T. L. (1980). <u>The PACE/DESIGN approach to solving problems</u>. Unpublished manuscript, Ohio University.

D'Zurilla, T. J., & Goldfried, M. R. (1971). Problem solving and behavior modification. <u>Journal of Abnormal Psychology, 78</u>, 107-126.

Mahoney, M. J. (1979). <u>Self-change: Strategies for solving personal problems</u>. New York: W. W. Norton & Company.

Manning, P. R., & DeBakey, L. (1987). <u>Medicine: Preserving the passion</u>. New York: Springer-Verlag.

Wheeler, D. D. & Janis, I. L. (1980). <u>A practical guide for making decisions</u>. New York: The Free Press.

THOUGHTS AND EMOTIONAL REACTIONS
VISUAL 6.1

CATASTROPHIZING

OVERGENERALIZATION

POLARIZED THINKING

FILTERING

<u>ASSERTIVENESS SKILLS</u>
VISUAL 6.2

AGGRESSIVE BEHAVIOR

PASSIVE BEHAVIOR

PASSIVE-AGGRESSIVE BEHAVIOR

ASSERTIVE BEHAVIOR

ROLE PLAYS

<u>SELECTING A PHYSICIAN</u>
VISUAL 6.3

RECORDS/BILLING PROCEDURES

PHYSICIAN AVAILABILITY

PHYSICIAN TRAINING

DRUG PRESCRIBING PRACTICES

PATIENT-DOCTOR RELATIONSHIP

SOLVED PROBLEMS EXERCISE
VISUAL 6.4

(1) <u>S</u>tate the problem.	
(2) <u>O</u>utline the problem.	
(3)<u>L</u>ist solutions. 　a.	(4)<u>V</u>iew the consequences. 　+
	-
b.	+
	-
c.	+
	-
d.	+
	-
e.	+
	-
f.	+
	-
(5)<u>E</u>xecute your solution.	
(6)<u>D</u>etermine if solution is effective.	

SOLVE FEELINGS EXERCISE
VISUAL 6.5

(1) <u>S</u> tate the problem.

(2) <u>O</u>bserve your thoughts.

(3) <u>L</u> ist your emotions.

(4) e<u>V</u> olve a coping attitude.

(5) <u>E</u> motional rescue!

SESSION SEVEN
REVIEW AND DISCUSSION

GOALS
1. Conclude the discussion of consequences of asthma.
2. Provide individual attention to participants with special problems or questions.
3. Process experiences with SOLVE Feelings and SOLVED Problems worksheets and behavior change attempts.
4. Promote continued use of social support as part of self-management efforts.

EQUIPMENT
Name tags.
Paper and pencils for all participants.
Overhead projector or slide projector.

SUPPLIES
Coffee, tea, snacks, or light lunch.

SESSION SEVEN OUTLINE

TOPIC/ ACTIVITY	REQUIRED MATERIAL	APPROXIMATE TIME ALLOWED
Welcome & introductions	Name tags	5 minutes
Questions about prior sessions/readings		10 minutes
Review SOLVE Feelings and SOLVED Problems worksheets		30-45 minutes
Consequences of asthma (as necessary)	See Session 5 (Visuals 5.1-5.7)	10-15 minutes
Open discussion and individual problem solving		15-35 minutes
Social support promotion	Pass a sheet for listing names and phone numbers	10 minutes

SESSION SEVEN TEACHING NOTES

Welcome and Salutations

Provide a name tag to each participant. Allow time for small talk among group members prior to getting into the session material.

Questions About Prior Sessions/Readings

Allow the group to ask questions about material covered earlier in the program.

Review of SOLVE Feelings and SOLVED Problems Worksheets

Encourage the participants to share their problem-solving efforts with the group, including both failures and successes. Reward all efforts with praise. Attempt to draw out participants' collective wisdom in solving asthma-related problems; the group will undoubtedly share some common problems. Allow the group to do as much of the problem solving as they can without leader feedback. Learning to generate potential solutions is more important than providing each participant with the one or two *best* solutions to their problem. Therefore, allow the group to generate several solutions before offering the obvious solution they may have missed.

Consequences of Asthma (continued if necessary)

Wrap up any discussion of asthma consequences which was first introduced in Session 5 (see Visuals 5.1-5.6). Encourage participants to share the consequences they have experienced in each category discussed (see Session 5). Rely on the Visuals to provide any information on consequences the group may fail to mention.

Open Discussion and Individual Problem Solving

This is the group's last chance to bring up special problems they are having with asthma management or coping with asthma sequelae. Group feedback and discussion, using the SOLVED Problems exercise as a framework, is recommended. The leader may choose to provide one-to-one time with individual participants at the conclusion of this last session. Clients with unremitting medical or psychological problems related to their asthma can be referred to an appropriate specialist.

Social Support Promotion

State the importance of social support in the workings of the Asthma Self-Management program and in the day to day self-management of asthma. Encourage the group to reveal the natural support systems they rely on (e.g., family, friends, church groups, others with asthma). Review step 4 in the asthma self-management steps: *seek the support of someone to help cope and make decisions about managing an unrelenting asthma attack*. Provide paper and pencils so participants can list their name and phone number if they wish to be available to others in the group as a support in asthma self-management. This commitment should be voluntary. It is understood that some participants will not wish to have their name on the list because of a spouse or other personal reason. The list can be xeroxed and shared with all those who provided their name and number.

A Note About the Authors

Thomas L. Creer has been a professor of psychology at Ohio University since 1980. Prior to that, he served for over a decade as the Director of the Behavioral Science Division at the National Asthma Center in Denver. He has spent almost a quarter of a century in investigating asthma and has published widely on the topic.

Harry Kotses, also a professor of psychology at Ohio University, has been investigating the psychophysiology of asthma for nearly two decades. He and Creer are the principal investigators for the research used as a basis for these handbooks.

Russ V. Reynolds, who is with the Department of Veterans' Affairs Medical Center in Charleston, South Carolina, received his doctorate from Ohio University in 1987. He has particular research interests in asthma and smoking cessation.